DIVINE HEALING 101

By
Dr Shaun Marler

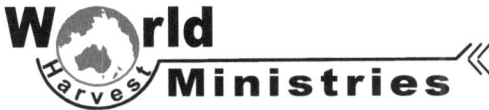

W⬤rld
Harvest Ministries

Harvesting The World For Jesus

Unless otherwise indicated, all scripture quotations are taken from the King James Version of the Bible.

Divine Healing 101
Copyright © 2020

Written by Dr Shaun Marler
Cover Design by Jay Binks & Sarah Freeman
Photo from Canva

Published by: World Harvest Ministries, PO Box 90, Bald Hills, Qld, 4036, Australia
whm.org.au

First Published November 2020

ISBN: 978-0-6485897-2-3

DEDICATION

I would like to dedicate this book to the great healing evangelists. Men and women of the Spirit that have impacted their
world for Christ. For their dedication to the Lord and His
Kingdom and tireless research and study of the scripture.
They have paved the way, leaving a legacy on which the Healers
of today can build. Their lives and testimonies of the wonderful works of God are an inspiration for this generation and the
generations still to come.

CHRIST IS COMPLETE IN YOU!

Foreword - Joshua Mills
Divine Healing 101

Too many people suffer unnecessarily for lack of knowledge.
I have seen this happen too often within the body of Christ,
and I have even personally witnessed this happening within my
own family. Quite a few years ago, my wife Janet and I went
to visit a relative that had been battling with several health
issues. Upon our arrival at their home, we offered to pray
for them and they gladly accepted our offer. In our prayer we
thanked God for their healing according to the finished work
that was accomplished on Calvary – we knew for sure in our
spirits that what God said in His Word was true. For us, the
healing had already been secured – but unfortunately, for our
relative – they didn't have the same revelation about healing.
Immediately following our time of prayer, they began speaking
about everything that was wrong in their body and everything
that was going to be wrong with their body. We were horrified!
It seemed like every word of blessing that we had spoken was
being cancelled by the words of cursing that were coming out
of our relative's mouth. You see, it's not that they were trying
to cancel the words we spoke – the issue was that they didn't
have the same revelation about healing that we did. The bible
tells us that whatever we speak will happen (see Mark 11:23).

You see, the power of both life and death are in our tongue (see Proverbs 18:21). Too many people have suffered at the lack of knowledge concerning God's healing promises. These promises are available to us... but we must make ourselves available to them!

For this reason, I am so thankful for this wonderful book that has been written by Dr. Shaun Marler. Divine Healing 101 offers us the knowledge of God's healing power through the personal testimonies, biblical examples and dynamic teaching of Dr. Marler. I agree with him when he states in this book "It is important to know the will of God concerning healing. After reading this book, you will clearly see that it is God's will for you to live your life in perfect health."

Understanding and receiving these truths from God's Word concerning healing will enable you to see yourself well, to know that sickness does not belong to you, and that you can live in the liberating healing grace of God each and every day of your life! I would encourage you to pick up several copies of this book and give them away to friends and family members that need a real touch from heaven. This book has the ability to become a miracle connection for those who read it.

Dr. Marler speaks from a life of experience. I have had the personal honor of spending time with him and his beautifully anointed family in Brisbane, Australia – and I have seen the way that he ministers in the power of the Spirit. Miracles are common... healing flows with ease... and the presence of God is experienced in a very real way. In this book, he offers you the keys, so that you can also begin moving in this same healing presence.

Prepare to embrace the abundant life – a life overflowing with healing for every area of need. And once you receive it, get ready to be used by God, as a minister of healing everywhere you go! This book will not only equip you with God's wisdom, but through the Spirit, it will also empower you with miraculous ability to heal the sick! Get ready to be trained in Divine Healing 101.

– Joshua Mills
Bestselling Author, Moving in Glory Realms & Power Portals
International Glory Ministries
London, Canada / Palm Springs, California
www.joshuamills.com

ACKNOWLEDGEMENTS

In preparing this book, I would like to acknowledge Dr. Steve Ryder, with whom I had the privileged of travelling around the world and learning first hand how to conduct healing crusades. I observed first hand, Steve ministering the Word of Knowledge and Gifts of Healing. I witnessed many thousands of miracles in great meetings in Africa, America, Australia and Europe.

I would also like to acknowledge Drummond Thom, Don Gossett and Dr. Lester Sumrall, with whom I fellowshipped many hours, gleaning from their vast experience in the healing ministry and international evangelism. They also shared with me insight into the lives of many of the great healing evangelists with whom they had personally worked with during their life long ministry journeys. Such men and women as Kathryn Kuhlman, William Freeman, A. A. Allen, William Branham, F.F. Bosworth, T.L. Osborne, John Osteen and many other of God's great generals.

A special acknowledgement to the writings of T.L. Osborne and F.F. Bosworth, from which I have made extensive studies and gleaned much while preparing this work.

THANK YOU

To everyone who has helped me prepare this book, from the original team, Peter Howlett, Marita Verdouw, Jay Binks and Elmarie Richards, who put together my mini book, 'Divine Healing Facts', I extend my gratitude and special thanks.

Now to Cherise Durham and Sarah Freeman for helping me bring this book to completion. Also to Kerrie, my wife and partner in this ministry, for her support and editing of this work.

Contents

DIVINE HEALING 101

INTRODUCTION

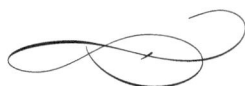

Over the past forty years of ministry whilst travelling the world, I have had the privilege of ministering divine healing to thousands of people. I have seen many people healed and set free from various ailments and diseases by praying the prayer of faith in the mighty name of Jesus.

In order to present the facts found in this book, I have gleaned from the teachings of many great men of God plus my own personal study and experience. My prayer is for you to open your heart and mind to God's plan of love and healing. You will then be able to join your faith and prayers with others to see their lives, free from pain, sickness and disease.

I have a great desire to see people healed and set free from sickness and pain. I want everyone to experience all the benefits provided for them by Jesus on the cross of Calvary.

I desire to empower people to win in life through Jesus Christ, with the signs He promised following them. Together let us love more, reach more, win more and do more for Jesus. Love and blessings, Shaun.

CHAPTER ONE

THE TRUTH SHALL SET YOU FREE

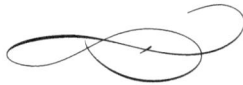

"And you shall know the truth, and the truth shall make you free." John 8:32

I believe all healing ultimately comes from God.

Many billions of dollars are spent each year around our world looking for the cures to new diseases. New viruses like Covid-19 are occurring, requiring constant discovery of new vaccines. More billions are being spent on mental health and mental illness problems now, than ever before in the history of mankind. All this to help aid and heal the pain and suffering of beautiful people who are afflicted one way or another.

"Jesus Christ the same yesterday, and to day, and for ever" Hebrews 13:8

The word of God reveals to us that we have an unseen enemy, Satan. Jesus told us in the gospel of John in chapter 10 and verse 10, that the thief (enemy) comes to steal, kill and destroy.

Jesus goes on to say that He has come, to reverse this, so that we may have life and have it in all its fullness and abundance.

Today many people believe that God can heal the sick but they have no personal knowledge of Jesus as the indwelling, ever present Healer. They have never studied the many facts which prove that physical health is part of every person's salvation.

They see other people healed, but they question whether healing is God's will for them. They are waiting for a special revelation of the will of God concerning their case. In the meantime, they are doing all they can, within the power of human skill, wisdom and knowledge, to receive it by the use of natural means. Through medical and scientific advances, people are looking for a cure, and there is nothing wrong with this! However it doesn't change the fact that it is God's will to heal them by divine means.

I encourage everyone to do all they can through medicine and natural therapies, if they need to, in order to relieve their suffering and pain. Yet it is still God's will for them to be healed, regardless whether they know it or not.

If it is not God's will for them to be well, it would be meaningless for them to seek recovery even through natural or medical means.

Because it is God's will for them to be healed and whole, then it is logical that the best way of recovery is by supernatural divine means. People can be supernaturally healed through the power and love of God, in the mighty Name of Jesus.

<u>The Bible Reveals the Will of God</u>

We also thank God that the Bible reveals the will of God in regard to the healing of the body as clearly as it reveals the will of God in regard to the saving of the soul. God does not have to give any special or individual revelation of His will, because He has plainly shown His revealed will in His Word (i.e. when the Bible declares He has promised to do it).

God has made many promises to heal. These promises are a revelation of His will. His Word (the Bible) is very clear regarding salvation. He desires everyone to become born again and receive His full salvation provided by Jesus. Likewise, the Word clearly reveals God's will regarding healing. God desires that everyone receives healing and lives a happy, healthy and prosperous life.

A careful study of the Scriptures by an unprejudiced person will clearly show that God is both the Saviour and the Healer of His people – it is always His will to save and to heal all those who are willing to serve Him. The contents of this book list 101 Biblical facts about divine healing.

It is suggested you read through this list often. Don't just leave it until you need healing, but read these facts over and over so that you can build your faith. The Word of God says that *"faith comes by hearing, and hearing by the word of God"*. Romans 10:17

Every revelation from God is designed to give you an encounter with God, for the specific purpose of lifting you to a higher plane of living.

_____

This is by no means saying that our medical systems are wrong. We thank God for doctors and modern medical break-throughs of today.

As you read these facts, faith will come into your spirit, so when you need faith for healing, faith in His Word will be there to draw upon. The Bible is full of simple steps to take in order to bring God's will into your life. It is very clear that God wants you prosperous in every area of your life. This includes your relationships, your mind, your spirit, your finances and your body. God can only ever give good things to you.

> *"Every good gift and every perfect gift is from above, and comes down from the Father of lights, with whom is no variableness, neither shadow of turning."* James 1:17

It is important to know the will of God concerning healing. After reading this book, you will clearly see that it is God's will for you to live your life in perfect health. As you gain this knowledge and understanding, you have taken the first step to receive your healing. You will be able to cast all doubt out of your mind and really know what God desires for you.

> *"Beloved, I wish above all things that you may prosper and be in health, even as your soul prospers."* 3 John 1:2

To prosper in your soul means to have knowledge, under-standing and stability in your thoughts, will and emotions. This book will help you to gain the knowledge and understanding of God's will regarding healing.

You will then be able to construct a positive mental picture of yourself completely healed in your mind and imagination.

The law of faith works by how we see ourselves. What we believe in our heart, see with the eyes of our faith and confess with our mouth, we will ultimately possess (some call this the law of attraction).

See yourself well, see yourself through the eyes of God and His word. See yourself as God sees you; healed and free through the finished works of Christ on the cross.

You can minister this truth to others, setting them free as well from the destructive works of the evil.

CHAPTER TWO

BRAIN TUMOURS HEALED

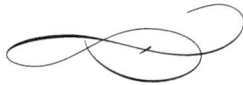

Over the years, I have prayed for many people that have received their healing miracles. Let me share with you two such testimonies.

Around 2005 my wife's best friend, Cheryl, whom she has known from her high school days, was diagnosed with a brain tumour. My wife had shared the Gospel with her many times, and Cheryl had already given her heart to Jesus.

At that time, I use to conduct a monthly healing service. On one of these Sunday night healing services, Cheryl and another friend brought a man along to be prayed for. Cheryl told me, that after I had ministered the scriptures and taught on healing, I called for people to come out for prayer. It was my practise to lay my hands upon them and ask God to heal their problems, releasing healing power and anointing into their bodies.

Cheryl came forward with the man who needed prayer. At the time, the church she attended didn't practise the laying on of hands for healing, so our kind of service was new for her.

When I asked Cheryl about how she received her healing, she explained it to me like this, "After you prayed for the man we had brought to the service, you said to me, "Is there anything you need from God?" To which, I replied to you, "Well, I have this lump in my head."

She then said that I got this strong look in my eye and she would never forget that look.

I asked her if I could lay hands upon her, to which she replied, "No, because I don't want to get pushed down." Cheryl explained to me that she had never been to a church where people fall over under the power of the Holy Spirit, and she thought that it was because they got pushed over. She said, "What happened next is that you placed your hand over my head, a few inches or centimetres in the air without touching my hair."

She told me that I got this strong look in my eyes, and I became angry at the devil and rebuked the spirit of infirmity that was empowering the tumour and causing it to grow in her head. She then said, that the last thing she remembers was that she felt heat and something was pulled out of the top of her head, and then she fell down. She laid on the floor, enjoying the warm feelings she was experiencing, which I later explained to her was the healing presence of God.

She had further MRI's and was scheduled for surgery. When the doctor performed the operation, he was able to make a very small incision in the top of her skull. The tumour that had been the size of a peach was now like a small pea, which as he explained to her, he just picked off from the membrane covering her brain, where it was loosely floating.

God had shrunk that growing tumour to the size of the pea, and it was literately sitting on the top of her brain. Cheryl told me that just like she felt when I prayed, it had been pulled out.

Now I share this testimony, to share with you another testimony of healing from a brain tumour. About five years ago, my wife Kerrie was experiencing, unexplained constant debilitating migraine headaches. She thought it had to do with her hormones and a combination of stress as a result of some circumstances we were facing at that time. However, after many months with these constant headaches, her Mum said, "You should visit my doctor." We were going to fly to Perth for a conference at the time but decided that it was best that Kerrie goes to the doctor first.

So we scheduled an appointment, and the doctor subsequently sent my wife for an MRI.

Now, just like her friend, Kerrie also was diagnosed with a brain tumour. When Kerrie picked up her CT scans, the receptionist said to Kerrie, "Good luck." She came home and said to me, "Shaun, I immediately put my trust in God, because I knew that when the receptionist said, good luck, the prognoses was not going to be good in the natural."

Kerrie was given six names of Brisbane's top neurosurgeons from which she had to pick one to go visit. We went to bed, prayed that by morning we would know which surgeon to call. When my wife woke up, one of the six names was at the forefront of her mind. She said to me, "Shaun, I know who I am going to call." She organized for her X-Ray's and scans to be sent to that doctor and rang the receptionist to make an appointment to see him. The receptionist said, "The Doctor is so busy, you won't get to see him for 6-8 weeks." My wife replied, "My doctor said, could you please just get him to look at the scans and test results." The receptionist replied, "Ok, but I cannot guarantee anything."

About an hour or so later, the receptionist called my wife and said, "The doctor would like to see you first thing in the morning." As you can imagine, we spent the night praying and thanking God for His goodness and healing power, that my wife's life was in the hands of God and we were believing for a good outcome.

The next morning, my wife went to the appointment, and the doctor said that he would have to operate within the next six days, otherwise in three weeks my wife could be dead. If she had any worse headaches in those six days, she was immediately to go straight back in. The brain tumour had grown so large it was, entwined behind her optic nerve and also stretching carotid artery. The carotid arteries are major blood vessels in the neck that supply blood to the brain, neck, and face. There are two carotid arteries, one on the right and one on the left. In the neck, each carotid artery branches into two divisions: The internal carotid artery supplies blood to the brain.

The internal carotid artery inside my wife's head was about to break. She would have then suffered a major brain bleed and died. Had we had flown to Perth, the pressure changes could have caused this artery to snap because of the size of the tumour. That night, when my wife came home, I prayed she would have no more headaches, and I laid hands on her and believed for a miracle. The headaches left that night and for the next six days, never returned.

I believe all healing is from God, and I am not opposed to medical intervention or medication. God wants His people well. God wants us to enjoy divine health and quality in life. In my wife's case, unlike her friend Cheryl, who, when I prayed, that tumour had shrunk, and a small pea sized lump was removed in about half an hour of surgery. My wife was going to have to undergo six hours of intensive surgery. People can ask, where is the healing? Well today, my wife and her friend Cheryl, enjoy a high quality of life, hold down jobs, spend time with their families and enjoy their grandchildren.

The doctor had given my wife only a 50% chance of surviving the surgery and a strong chance of her losing some abilities. Instead, he told me, after the surgery that the brain tumour had come away nicely. When I first found out that my wife in six days' time, would undergo surgery, I immediately prayed. In my prayer, I thanked the Lord that the tumour would be removed nicely, with no ongoing battles. I thanked God that the surgery would be a total success. After the surgery was complete, my wife was taken to the recovery ward. The surgeon, who had performed the operation, came and spoke to me. He said, "That she is not completely out of the woods yet." He went on to say that he was able to remove it all, even from the nerves behind the eye. In the removal, nothing was damaged. Today Kerrie has great vision, enjoys long walks, drives her car and has now been given the all clear.

You can't tell that her skull was cut open from one side to the other. You wouldn't even know, talking with her that she ever had, this tumour and major brain surgery.

I have seen many people instantly healed as I have prayed, but in these two testimonies, both these ladies went through a different journey during their miracle. Both have received their healing miracles, and further MRI's have shown no re-growth of any tumours.

Even though Kerrie and Cheryl had different measures of medical intervention, they both testify that their healings are miracles from God. They thank God for the doctors, but know that without God's miracle-working power and the prayers of-fered on their behalf, they probably would not be here today.

Praise God, our God is the healer God. He wants you whole and well. I encourage you to read this book, and whenever you or a loved one or someone you know needs a miracle,you can stand on and declare the promises in God's word. Many of which, I have revealed in this teaching.

Lay hands on the sick, by faith in the name of Jesus and the sick will get well, recover and be made whole.

When I lay hands on people, sometimes they fall down (in the Spirit), and sometimes they don't. It depends on how the Spirit and anointing are flowing and working at that time of prayer. It can also depend on how God is leading the person, in this case me, to work the miracle. The healing is not about whether a person falls down or doesn't fall down. It is about re-leasing faith in the name of Jesus for the miracle. Remember, it is the name of Jesus and faith in that name that causes the healing to manifest in the persons life that is being prayed for.

"Jesus Christ is the same yesterday, today and forever." Hebrews 13:8

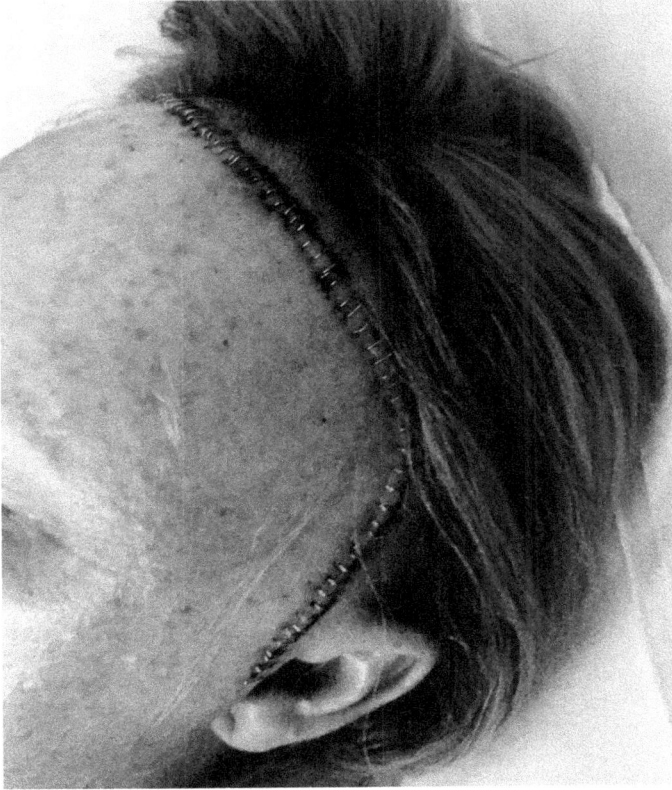

*Kerrie is forever grateful for God's goodness, and the wonderful surgeon and doctors that performed her brain surgery. In this picture you can see the stainless steal surgical staples, used in the surgery. There was too many to count. Kerrie knows that without God's healing hand, through the whole procedure, she would not be here today to tell her testimony. *Refer to Footnotes.*

CHAPTER THREE

HEALING

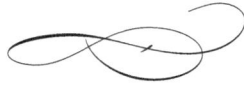

God is a Healer

God revealed Himself to the people of Israel as a healer-God. Jehovah Rapha. He promised to keep disease from them if they would obey His Word.

> *"If you will diligently hearken to the voice of the Lord thy God, and wilt do that which is right in His sight, and wilt give ear to His commandments, and keep all His statutes, I will put none of these diseases upon thee, which I have brought upon the Egyptians; for I am the Lord that heals you."* (Exodus 15:26 Old Testament.)

Healing - One of God's Benefits

God is a Father to His children. Because of His compassion for those He loves, He has made provision for their healing. This is one of the benefits of having a loving heavenly Father who cares for our every need.

"Bless the Lord. O my soul, and forget not all His benefits: Who forgives all your iniquities; who heals all your diseases". (Psalms 103:2,3 Old Testament).

Notice that forgiveness is one of God's benefits. They are both placed together in this passage of scripture. God is concerned about both our spiritual healing and our physical healing.

Messiah Suffers for Our Healing

The prophet Isaiah wrote about the One who was to suffer, the Messiah or Redeemer of Israel. He was writing about Jesus taking our punishment for our sins. Jesus suffered for us in every way we deserved to suffer. Physically, mentally, spiritually. He did it in order that we might not have to suffer these things. He was our substitute, our Saviour.

The four Gospel writers tell us what they **SAW** and **HEARD** about the suffering of Christ. On the other hand, Isaiah tells us what was **REVEALED** to him by the Spirit of God concerning Christ's sufferings.

*"Surely He has borne our griefs and carried our sorrows; yet we did esteem Him stricken, smitten of God, and afflicted. But He was wounded for our transgressions, He was bruised for our iniquities; the chastisement of our peace was upon Him; and **WITH HIS STRIPES WE ARE HEALED.** All we like sheep have gone astray; we have turned every*

one to his own way; and the Lord has laid on Him the iniquity of us all" (Isaiah 53:4-6 Old Testament).

The two words *"griefs"* and *"sorrows"* in the first phrase of the passage could equally be translated sicknesses and pains. This will be clearer after reading Matthew 8:16-17. From these three verses, we see the variety of things Jesus suffered as He took our place and God's judgement for sin fell on Him.

He Took Our Infirmities and Bore Our Sicknesses

While Jesus walked the face of the earth, He ministered healing to every part of man. He cast out devils, healed the sick, forgave sin, and restored wholeness to those tormented by Satan. In recording these events, Matthew quoted from Isaiah 53:4 (Old Testament) concerning the substitutionary work of Christ.

"When the evening was come they brought unto Him many that were possessed with devils; and He cast out the spirits with His Word, and healed all that were sick; that it might be fulfilled which was spoken by Isaiah the prophet, saying, **HE HIMSELF TOOK OUR INFIRMITIES, AND BARE OUR SICKNESS"** *(*Matthew 8:16-17).

Not only did He take our infirmities and bare all our sicknesses on the cross, but also during His ministry, He relieved people of infirmities and sicknesses. He did this in relation to sins also. Not only did He take our sins on the cross, but He also forgave men of their sins before the crucifixion.

Healed by His Stripes

Peter was a man who witnessed the mock trial of Jesus. He was well acquainted with the happenings on Calvary. He wrote about the effects that Jesus' suffering would have on our lives. He mentions both the spiritual and the physical results of Christ's atonement.

> *"Who His own self bare our sins in His own body on the tree, that we, being dead to sins, should live unto righteousness: **BY WHOSE STRIPES YOU ARE HEALED"*** 1 Peter 2:24.

The phrase *"by whose stripes you are healed"* is a direct reference to Isaiah 53:5 in the Old Testament. You remember that Jesus was scourged or whipped before his crucifixion (Mark 15:15). The physical punishment that He took was for our healing, for *"with His stripes we are healed"* (Isaiah 53:5). All the punishment Jesus received before and during the crucifixion was for our healing - spirit, soul and body.

Satan is the Author of Sickness and Disease

Before Adam's sin in the garden, there was no sin or death on the earth. After his disobedience, sin and death with all of their evil companions (hatred, bitterness, jealously, sickness, disease, torment) entered into the world (Romans 5:12). Jesus was sent to re-establish the wholeness that man had before the fall. He was the Redeemer, the One sent to buy us back from the dominion of Satan. Jesus freed the people who were captive to Satan's devices. He healed the sick, delivered the oppressed, opened prison doors, and preached the Good News.

"How God anointed Jesus of Nazareth with the Holy Spirit and with power: who went about doing good, and healing all that were oppressed of the devil: for God was with Him." (Acts 10:38).

This scripture, as well as all four gospels, clearly reveals that the devil oppresses people with sickness, and Jesus heals people who are sick. Never confuse these two. God desires an abundant life for us, and the devil wants to steal, to kill and to destroy. (John 10:10)

God Wants Us In Health

"Beloved, I wish above all things that you may prosper and be in health, even as your soul prospers" (3 John 2).

God is interested in our health, spiritually and physically. He wants our bodies to be just as free from Satan's influence as He does our hearts.

"For you are bought with a price: therefore glorify God in your body, and in your spirit, which are God's" (1 Corinthians 6:20).

Not only are we to live holy and pure lives in our body, but also it is possible for us to live in health. We have been bought with the blood of Christ. The price has been paid for spiritual and physical health.

Redeemed From the Curse

"Christ hath redeemed us from the curse of the law, being made a curse for us: for it is written, Cursed is every one that hangs on a tree: That the blessing of Abraham might come on the Gentiles through Jesus Christ; that we might receive the promise of the Spirit through faith" (Galatians 3:13-14).

There was a curse pronounced upon those who would not keep God's laws (Deuteronomy 28:15-68). This curse generally included poverty, sickness, and death. Since all men were sinners, there was no man who could fully keep all God's laws (Romans 3:23).

Jesus entered the earth as a man and lived His life without sin. As he hung on the cross, He was actually made to be a curse for us, as our substitute. He took the curse we deserved. He took our poverty, our sickness, and our death (sin), so that we might receive the blessings God has promised to Abraham and those keeping His law. These include an abundant supply for every need in our lives (Deuteronomy 28:1-14 Old Testament).

In Acts 10:38 it tells us, *"How God anointed Jesus of Nazareth with the Holy Ghost and with power: who went about doing good, and healing all that were oppressed of the devil; for God was with him."*

Here we can see it was God who anointed Jesus with Holy Spirit power to do good and to heal. Jesus Christ came to save the lost and heal the sick. From the above scripture, we can also determine that sickness is an oppression sent by Satan from the kingdom of darkness.

Jesus is Still the Same

"Jesus Christ the same yesterday, and today, and forever" (Hebrews 13:8). The reason Jesus healed people was because of His compassion. He saw their needs and met them. He is still the same. His compassion has not stopped. He loves us just as much as He did those in the time of His earthly ministry. His power is not stopped just because He is no longer visibly in our midst. His power and effectiveness are even greater today because He can be present in all places at all times by His Spirit. *"His mercy endures forever"* (Psalm 136 in the Old Testament).

Prayer of Faith - Anointing with Oil

We know from the book of Acts that the healing ministry of Christ did not stop with His death and resurrection. It continued through the twelve disciples and the other believers (Mark 16:15-19).

There were numerous ways in which people received healing under Jesus' ministry. Today men can receive healing from the basis of numerous passages of scripture. These include: Mark 11:22-24; John 16:23-24; Matthew 18:18-20; Mark 16:18; James 5:14-15; Exodus 15:26; Psalms 103:3; 1 Peter 2:24; Matthew 8:16-17.

One important method is anointing with oil and praying the prayer of faith. It demonstrates to us that God's power can be ministered by believers, and this shows that healing did not end when Christ died or when the apostles died. Healing is still provided for us today.

> *"Is any sick among you? Let him call for the elders of the church, and let them pray over him, anointing him with oil in the name of the Lord: and the prayer of faith shall save the sick, and the Lord shall raise him up; and if he have committed sins, they shall be forgiven him"* (James 5:14-15).

<u>Laying on of Hands</u>

Mark 16:15-18 states, *"And he said unto them, 'Go you into all the world, and preach the gospel to every creature. He that believes and is baptised shall be saved; but he that believes not shall be dammed. And these signs shall follow them that believe; In my name shall they cast out devils; they shall speak with new tongues; They shall take up serpents; and if they drink any deadly thing, it shall not hurt them; they shall lay hands on the sick, and they shall recover."*

Here in verse 18, we can see that Jesus said we can lay hands on the sick in His name, and they would recover or get well. Laying on of hands is another way by which healing can be received.

I have ministered the word in many countries of the earth including, the Philippines, in Australia, in Czechoslovakia,

India, Canada, South Africa, Sierra Leone, Malawi, Zambia, Zimbabwe, USA, Solomon Islands, Kenya, Ethiopia, Vanuatu, Papua New Guinea, Fiji, Samoa etc. After people have heard and believed the Word of God, I have personally laid hands on thousands of people, and in the name of Jesus, seen many hundreds healed as God's power flowed out through my hands and into their bodies.

Not all these healings were instantaneous, although many were, yet many from that point of contact began to recover and get well. I have seen legs grow longer and people throw down their walking sticks, as God's power flowed through their bodies and healed them. **Remember, "Jesus is the same yesterday, today and forever"** Hebrews 13:8.

> *"Therefore, leaving the principles of the doctrine of Christ, let us go unto perfection; not laying again the foundations of repentance from dead works, and of faith toward God, of the doctrine of baptisms, and of laying on of hands, and of resurrection of the dead, and of eternal judgment" (Hebrews 6:1&2).*

Here we see in the Book of Hebrews, that the doctrine of laying on of hands that Jesus taught, is listed as a foundation principle that all believers should know before they can go on to maturity (perfection) in the body of Christ.

Many churches believe in baptism, but leave out the doctrine of laying on of hands, yet we can see here the two go hand in hand. The minds of men in these last days have deleted many of the doctrines of Christ from their church services, and because of this, they are not seeing the power of God in manifestation.

_____

Any doctrine that cannot be substantiated by scripture and verse is wrong and is from the minds of men.

All doctrine must be backed up by the word of God taken in context with the chapter from where it came.

Let me bring a warning from the Bible:

> *"Now the Spirit speaks expressly, that in the latter times some shall depart from the faith, giving heed to seducing spirits, and doctrines of devils."* (1 Timothy 4:1)

The devil tells man's mind that it is okay to take things out of the Bible and say they are not for today. But it isn't. It is wrong to delete doctrines that will set men free; it is wrong not to preach and teach the truth, because the truth in God's Word when revealed, sets men free.

The devil wants you to be sick and die, but God wants you to be well and prosper even as your soul prospers (3 John 2).

God tells us in Exodus 15:26, *"I am the Lord that heals you."* He will release His mighty power to work in and through us as we obey Him and lay our hands on people to see them healed.

> *"Till I come, give attendance to reading, to exhortation, to doctrine. Neglect not the gift that is in thee, which was given thee by prophecy, with the laying on of the hands of the presbytery."* (1 Timothy 4:13 & 14)

Here Paul told Timothy to give attention to doctrine, and not to neglect the gift that was given him by the laying on of hands. Healing and laying on of hands is a doctrine (teaching) of the early Christian church. This has not changed. Jesus is still the same, and He still heals and gives us the power to do this work through His name.

Power to Heal

The power of God will flow through anyone's hands if they are a believer and take God at His Word, and in faith, lay their hands on the sick in the name of Jesus.

You are a candidate for the power of God to flow through your hands to heal the sick. You can begin in faith by praying for your own family and friends and laying hands on them (with their permission, of course) to see them recover and get well.

Casting Out Devils

Another way to heal the sick is by casting out a devil or spirit of infirmity. In verse 17 of Mark 16 (previously mentioned), Jesus said we have the power to cast devils in His name.

This is any devil or spirit that is causing the curse to be active in your life. Many times the problems we are facing or going through are caused by devils or demons in the unseen realm of the spirit working through the curse of the law against us. Their destructive influences can be felt or seen in many ways.

In many of the different countries and places of the world that I have ministered, the Lord has instructed me to bind the evil forces of darkness first. On the prayer lines, I have prayed for hundreds of people over the years, taking authority over the spirit of infirmity in their life or body. That is the evil spirit that is empowering the sickness to destroy them. I have spoken to the spirit, casting it out and telling it to leave the person.

I have observed that as the spirit of infirmity and sickness has left, healing relief and deliverance has flowed back into their lives.

Take Authority

Now before I pray, I always bind the spirit of infirmity over the life of the person I am praying for. I cast out the spirit, telling it that it has no more power over that individual's life because of the shed blood and authority of the name of Jesus. I remind the spirit, that is causing the sickness to manifest in the person's body, that it was defeated by Jesus Christ at Calvary.

I then command the sickness to leave the person's body, demanding the part causing them pain to be made whole, healed and function normally how God created it to function.

It is Jesus who works with us to confirm the word, with signs following.

Chapter Four

Why Healing Is Important

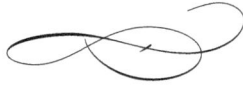

"The thief comes only to steal, and to kill, and to destroy: I am come that they might have life, and that they might have it more abundantly." John 10:10

One of the main areas that the thief steals from us is in the area of our health. There are many problems that are associated with sickness. It robs us of our time, it robs us of our money, and it robs us of our relationships, by destroying quality time with our family and friends.

In simple terms, we can see that sickness will nullify your capabilities, and prevent you from progressing and helping in the kingdom of God. Our taxes are being channelled into multi-national companies, just to keep abreast of disease control and to supply medication.

In this day and age, some Christian leaders tell us that physical healing belongs to the past. However, healing was an important part of the ministry of Jesus while he was on earth, and Divine Healing is one of the promises of God. When believed and acted upon, any promise of God is transformed into the power of God.

"For they are life unto those that find them, and health to all their flesh." **Proverbs 4:22**

The Word of God is full of his promises to us, and it is our responsibility to discover them, to believe them, and to act upon them.

To fully know God, we must know Him as the Healer - otherwise, we are missing a major dimension of our relationship with him.

Exodus 15:26 *"...For I am the Lord that heals you."*

It is extremely important to realize that divine healing is God's will. John was inspired by the Holy Spirit to write in III John 2 *"Beloved, I wish above all things that you may prosper and be in health, even as thy soul prospers."*

It was important to Jesus to do the will of the Father, and he went about healing the people.

"I come to do your will, O God." Hebrews 10:7

"For I came down from heaven, not to do mine own will, but the will of him that sent me." John 6:38

"And Jesus went about all the cities and villages, teaching in their synagogues, and preaching the gospel of the kingdom, and healing every sickness and every disease among the people." Matthew 9:35

The anointing of the Holy Spirit is a very important part of Healing. In Luke chapter 4, verse 18, we read about how the Holy Spirit anointed Jesus:

"The Spirit of the Lord is upon me, because he has anointed me to preach the Gospel to the poor; he has sent me to heal the broken hearted, to preach deliverance to the captives, and recovering of sight to the blind, to set at liberty them that are bruised."

In Acts 10:38 we read, *"How God anointed Jesus of Nazareth with the Holy Ghost and with power: who went about doing good, and healing all that were oppressed of the devil; for God was with him."*

It was the power of the Holy Spirit that healed people.

Healing was an important part of the ministry of Jesus:

As we follow Jesus through the New Testament, we find him ministering healing in many different situations. His compassion for the sick was constantly evident.

"And when Jesus was come into Peter's house, he saw his wife's mother laid, and sick of a fever. And he touched her hand, and the fever left her: and she arose, and ministered unto them. When the even was come, they brought unto him many that were possessed with devils: and he cast out the spirits with His Word, and healed all that were sick: That it might be fulfilled which was spoken by Isaiah the prophet saying, He took our infirmities, and bare our sicknesses." Matthew 8:14-17

Healing was an important part of the training and ministry of Jesus' Disciples and followers:

"And when he had called unto him his twelve disciples, he gave them power against unclean spirits, to cast them out, and to heal all manner of sickness and all manner of disease. And as ye go, preach, saying, The kingdom of heaven is at hand. Heal the sick, cleanse the lepers, raise the dead, cast out devils: freely ye have received, freely give." Matthew 10:1, 7 - 8

Jesus wanted all believers to heal the sick. When he sent out the seventy-two, he instructed them to heal the sick.

"After these things the Lord appointed seventy others also, and sent them two by two before His face into every city and place where He Himself was about to go.... And heal the sick who are there, and say to

them, The kingdom of God has come near to you."
Luke 10:1, 9

Healing is important if we are to be obedient, and do the works of Jesus: Our Lord Jesus Christ says that we will perform healings and miracles just like him:

"Most assuredly, I say to you, he who believes in Me, the works that I do he will do also; and greater works than these he will do, because I go to the Father."
John 14:12

Healing can save your life and the lives of your family and friends. Healing in our body is a provision of God for us.

"I shall not die, but live, and declare the works of the Lord." Psalms 118:17

"Is there anyone among you sick? Let him call for the elders of the church, and let them pray over him, anointing him with oil in the name of the Lord."
James 5:14

If we do not minister healing to the sick, then the suffering that Christ bore on his body was in vain:

"But he was wounded for our transgressions, He was bruised for our iniquities; the chastisement for our peace was upon Him, and by His stripes we are healed." Isaiah 53:5

"I do not set aside the grace of God; for if righteousness comes through the law, then Christ died in vain." Galatians 2:21

Ministering healing by the laying on of hands is an important part of the great commission that Jesus left all believers.

"If you love me, keep my commandments." John 14:15

The great commission gives us a directive to preach the good news. This includes the good news that God is our healer:

"And He said to thee, Go into all the world and preach the gospel to every creature. He who believes and is baptized will be saved; but he who does not believe will be condemned. And these signs will follow those who believe: In My name they will cast out demons; they will speak with new tongues." The last part of verse 18 declares, "That they will lay hands on the sick and the sick will recover." Mark 16:15-18

Healing confirms God's Word to a lost and dying world. The world today needs Jesus. God has commissioned us to go with signs and wonders following to confirm his word. Healing the sick will help people to open their eyes to the truth of the gospel.

CHAPTER FIVE

WHERE DOES SICKNESS COME FROM

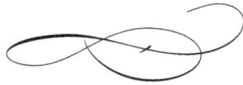

In order to be enlightened on how to deal with sickness, we have to understand its origin, source and purpose. Is sickness from God or from Satan? If there is any doubt in our mind, our faith will be ineffective.

> *"But of the tree of the knowledge of good and evil, thou shalt not eat of it: for in the day that thou eatest thereof thou shalt surely die."* Genesis 2:17

> *"Every good gift and every perfect gift is from above, and comes down from the Father of lights, with whom there is no variableness, neither shadow of turning."* James 1:17

A question is often asked, "Is sickness one of the ways that God works things together for our good?" *"All things work together for good to them that love God.."* (Romans 8:28 KJV)

This is often quoted to attempt to show that sickness is one of these "all things" that work together for good. More accurate translations give us a clearer understanding of this scripture. From the NIV Romans 8:28 says;

"We know that in all things God works for the good of those who love him, who have been called according to his purpose."

We see here the emphasis is ***"in all things"*** God works for our good. If we are sick, God works with us for our healing.

Another question that is often asked, "Is being sick one of the ways that we are to "suffer for him?" Philippians 1:29 says;

"For unto you it is given in the behalf of Christ, not only believe on him, but also to suffer for his sake."

To avoid misinterpreting this scripture, it is necessary to consider the setting and subject of discussion. In this case, Paul is in prison, writing about his suffering for the faith of the gospel, and about the Philippians suffering for the sake of the gospel. It is very clear that the suffering Paul is writing about is because of opposition to salvation by faith in Jesus Christ. This suffering was not related to sickness in any way.

This brings us to the question, "Is it God's will to be sick?" No, it is God's will that we live in divine health.

"Beloved, I wish above all things that you may prosper and be in health, even as your soul prospers." 3 John 2

Does God put sickness on people to correct, discipline, or punish them?

No, it is Satan and not God, who is the one who puts sickness and disease on people. Job 2:7 says, *"So Satan went forth from the presence of the Lord, and smote Job with sore boils from the sole of his foot unto his crown."*

Is God the Source of Sickness? No, **the Father calls sickness captivity.**

> *"And the Lord turned the captivity of Job, when he prayed for his friends: also the Lord gave Job twice as much as he had before."* Job 42:10

The Bible describes Job's healing as deliverance from captivity.

Jesus calls sickness bondage.

> *"And ought not this woman, being a daughter of Abraham, whom Satan hath bound, lo, these eighteen years, be loosed from this bond on the sabbath day?"* Luke 13:16

- For eighteen years, the woman had a crippling, arthritic type disease that kept her bent over and unable to stand erect.
- Jesus dealt with the source 'a spirit of infirmity' that Satan had assigned to put her in bondage. (Verse 11)
- Jesus laid his hands on her as He cast out the spirit of infirmity, "Woman, thou art loosed from thine infirmity." (verse 12)

The Holy Spirit calls sickness oppression.

"Jesus...went about doing good, and healing all that were oppressed of the devil." Acts 10:38

• Oppression or sickness is not from God - it is of the devil.
• The ministry of Jesus was 'to let the oppressed free'. (Isaiah 58:6)

Each person of the Godhead expressed themselves regarding sickness and disease. The Father called sickness captivity. The Son called sickness bondage. The Holy Spirit called sickness oppression.

Jesus sets the captive free - all bondages, including those of sickness and infirmity, could never be God's will. Jesus was anointed by the Holy Spirit *"to set at liberty them that are bruised."* (Luke 4:18)

"Is not this the fast that I have chosen? To loose the bonds of wickedness, to undo the heavy burdens, and to let the oppressed go free, and that you break every yoke?" Isaiah 58:6

To know Jesus and His truth is to be set free from bondage.

"And you shall know the truth, and the truth shall make you free." John 8:32

"Jesus is, "the way, the truth and life." John 14:6

Does sickness bring glory to God? Is sickness a blessing or a curse? Obviously, sickness is a curse, and does not bring glory to God.

Sickness is from Satan.

Satan and his angels were cast down to earth after their rebellion in heaven.

> "And there was war in heaven: Michael and his angels fought against the dragon and the dragon fought and his angels, And prevailed not; neither was their place found any more in heaven. And the great dragon was cast out, that old serpent, called the Devil, and Satan, which deceiveth the whole world: he was cast out into the earth, and his angels were cast out with him. And I heard a loud voice saying in heaven, Now is come salvation, and strength, and the kingdom of our God, and the power of his Christ: for the accuser of our brethren is cast down, which accused them before our God day and night." Revelation 12:7-10

Man was created in God's image sometime after Satan's fall. Man was created:

- To look like God
- To walk like God
- To talk like God
- To rule over this earth

"...Let us make man in our image, after our likeness: and let them have dominion over the fish of the sea, and over the fowl of the air, and over the cattle and over all the earth, and over every creeping thing that creeps upon the earth." Genesis 1:26, 28

When Satan saw humans, looking like God, his hatred was turned against humanity:

"The thief comes only to steal, and to kill, and to destroy." John 10:10

Loss, death, and destruction are always the work of Satan. For four thousand years after the fall in the Garden of Eden, man lived under the captivity and bondage of the devil.

• Men and women created in God's image now had the features of their faces, and their bodies eaten away with leprosy.
• Human beings who had been created to walk in dominion were crippled, blind, and begging on the roadside.

Jesus said, "I have come that they may have life, and that they may have it more abundantly." John 10:10

THE SOURCE OF ALL SICKNESS AND DISEASE IS SATAN - NOT GOD!

CHAPTER SIX

101 DIVINE HEALING FACTS
(Taken from the writings of T.L. Osborn and
F. F. Bosworth. Revised and expanded).

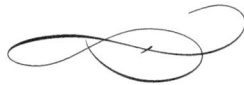

Healing as revealed in God's Word

1. Sickness is no more natural than sin, but a result of man's rebellion to God's laws. In the beginning, God made all things *"very good"* (Genesis 1:31). Therefore, we should not look for the cure of sin nor of sickness in the natural, but from God. We were created happy, strong, healthy, prosperous, and in fellowship with our God. Until the fall of mankind happened and we fell from this place of higher living. We now need to repent, change our way of thinking and follow God's plan, on how to live and divine health will follow.

2. Because sin and sickness both came into the world through man's rebellion in the garden of Eden. It would now take the obedience of one man, Jesus Christ, to set us free. From the bible, we can see that sickness is a result of sin.

Therefore, we must look for the healing of both sin and sickness in the Saviour, Jesus Christ, who restores us from the fall that occurred in the garden of Eden.

> *"Wherefore, as by one man sin entered into the world, and death by sin; and so death passed upon all men, for that all have sinned."* Romans 5:12

3. When Jesus Christ died on the Cross of Calvary, He not only paid the price for our sins, but He paid the price for our sicknesses as well.

> *"Surely he hath borne our griefs, and carried our sorrows: yet we did esteem him stricken, smitten of God, and afflicted. But he was wounded for our transgressions, he was bruised for our iniquities: the chastisement of our peace was upon him; and with his stripes we are healed."* Isaiah 53:4-5

4. God made a covenant of healing with His children (the Israelites) when he called them out of Egypt. Throughout their history, as a result of their rebellion to God's laws, they ended up in sickness, trouble and disease. Every time they turned to God in repentance (asking for forgiveness and turning away from their sin) through confession (speaking out their sins); we can see that, when their sins were forgiven, their sicknesses were healed. God forgave them of their sins and healed them of their sicknesses.

"And said, If you will diligently hearken to the voice of the LORD your God, and will do that which is right in his sight..... for I am the LORD that heals you." Exodus 15:26

"And you shall serve the LORD your God, and he shall bless your bread, and your water; and I will take sickness away from the midst of you." Exodus 23:25

5. In Numbers 21:8, We can see an awesome miracle take place. The people had been bitten by poisonous snakes in the wilderness. This would result in their death, but as they looked at a brazen serpent on a pole, God healed them.

"And the LORD said unto Moses, Make thee a fiery serpent, and set it upon a pole: and it shall come to pass, that every one that is bitten, when he looks upon it, shall live." Number 21:8 (See also Numbers 21:4 – 9)

This was a representation of what was to happen on the cross with Jesus. *"And as Moses lifted up the serpent in the wilderness, even so (for the same purpose) must the Son of man be lifted up: That whosoever believes in him should not perish, but have eternal life."* John 3:14-15

The people cried to God in Moses time, and He heard their cry and provided a miracle solution.
– the serpent lifted up. Those who cry to God today discover that God has heard their cry and has provided them with a

remedy – Christ lifted up. If everyone who looked at the brazen serpent was healed then, it is logical that everyone who looks at Jesus can be healed today.

Since their curse was removed by the lifting up of the "type of Christ", or representation of Calvary (the pole), our curse was certainly removed by Calvary itself, as Jesus Christ hung upon the cross for us.

> *"Christ has redeemed us from the curse of the law, being made a curse for us: for it is written, Cursed is every one that hangs on a tree."* Galatians 3:13

6. The people had sinned against God in the times of Moses. Still to this day, people sin against God's laws. Sickness is a result of sin (see Romans 5:12), so if we deal with the sin problem, then the sickness can also be dealt with. In Moses' time, people repented of their ways and turned to the serpent lifted up. So too today, we need to repent of our sins against God and turn to Jesus, who is lifted up.

7. The poisonous serpent-bite resulted in death then, just like the wages of sin today still results in death. Romans 6:23 says *"For the wages of sin is death; but the gift of God is eternal life (rich, blessed and everlasting) through Jesus Christ our Lord."*

8. The remedy back then was for *"every one that is bitten"* (see Numbers 21:8). The remedy today is for *"whosoever believes."*

"For God so loved the world, that he gave his only begotten Son, THAT WHOSOEVER BELIEVES in him should not perish, but have everlasting life." John 3:16

There were no exceptions in Moses' time – their remedy was for "every one that is bitten." There are no exceptions to-day – our remedy is for "whosoever believes."

9. In their remedy, they received both forgiveness for their sins and healing for their bodies.

"If we confess our sins, he is faithful and just to forgive us our sins, and to cleanse us from all unrighteousness." 1 John 1:9

10. Everyone was commanded to do his own looking at the remedy then. Everyone is commanded to do his own believing in Christ today.

"That whosoever believes in him should not perish, but have eternal life." John 3:15

"Ask, and it shall be given you; seek, and ye shall find; knock, and it shall be opened unto you." Mathew 7:7

11. The people did not need to beg nor make an offering to God then. There was only one condition: *"When he looks...."* We do not need to beg or make an offering to Christ today. There is only one condition: *" Whosoever believes."*

12. They were not told to look to Moses, but rather to the remedy then. We are not told to look to the preacher or any other person, but to Jesus Christ today.

> *"Keep yourselves in the love of God, looking for the mercy of our Lord Jesus Christ unto eternal life."* Jude 1:21

> *"Looking unto Jesus, the author and finisher of our faith."* Hebrews 12:2

The people were not to look to the symptoms of their snake-bites then, but rather to the remedy. We are not to look to the symptoms of our sins and diseases today, but to our remedy, Jesus Christ.

> *"Then look up, and lift up your heads; for your redemption draws nigh."* Luke 21:28

13. 'Everyone that is bitten, when he looks upon it, shall live', was the promise to all then, without exception. *'Whosoever believes in Him should not perish, but have everlasting life'*, is the promise to all today, without exception. (see John 3:16)

14. The "type" of Calvary could not mean more to those Israelites then than Calvary means to us today. Today we can receive more blessings through the actual Calvary than the Israelites received through the 'type' of Calvary.

"How shall we escape (flee from), if we neglect so great salvation (rescue, safety, deliver, healing, saved); which at the first began to be spoken by the Lord, and was confirmed unto us by them that heard him." Hebrews 2:3

15. God revealed Himself to Hezekiah as the Healer of the people.

"Turn again, and tell Hezekiah the captain of my people, Thus saith the LORD, the God of David thy father, I have heard thy prayer, I have seen thy tears: behold, I will heal thee: on the third day thou shalt go up unto the house of the LORD." 2 Kings 20:5

16. God continually healed people throughout the Bible. It is recorded many times that when the Lord was asked for healing, He healed those that asked.

"So Abraham prayed unto God: and God healed Abimelech, and his wife, and his maidservants; and they bare children." Genesis 20:7

"And Moses cried unto the LORD, saying, Heal her now, O God, I beseech you." Numbers 12:13

"Thus says the LORD, the God of David your father, I have heard your prayer, I have seen your tears: behold, I will heal you:" 2 Kings 20:5

"And the LORD hearkened to Hezekiah, and healed the people." 2 Chronicles 30:20

"O LORD my God, I cried unto You, and You have healed me." Psalm 30:2

17. Israel (God's chosen people) knew God as their Healer and the one who blessed them (empowered them to prosper).

"And he will love you, and bless you, and multiply you: he will also bless the fruit of your womb, and the fruit of your land, your corn, and your wine, and your oil, the increase of your kine, and the flocks of your sheep, in the land which he sware unto your fathers to give you. You shall be blessed above all people: there shall not be male or female barren among you, or among your cattle. And the LORD will take away from you all sickness, and will put [permit] none of the evil diseases of Egypt, which you know, upon you...." Deuteronomy 7:13-15

Today we are God's chosen people. He remains our Healer.

"But you are a chosen generation, a royal priesthood, a holy nation, a peculiar people; that you should show forth the praises of him who has called you out of darkness into his marvellous light." 1 Peter 2:9

18. One of the benefits of knowing the Lord is healing.

"Bless the LORD, O my soul, and forget not all his benefits: Who forgives all my iniquities; who heals all my diseases." Psalm 103:2-3

19. In Psalm 91, God promises protection for our bodies as well as for our souls, if we abide in Him. In the New Testament, John wishes *"above all things that you may prosper and be in health, even as your soul prospers"* 3 John 2

Both scriptures show that God's will is that we be healthy in our bodies as we are in our souls. It is never God's will for our souls to be sick. It is never God's will for our bodies to be sick. Read Psalm 91 to understand God's will regarding your health.

"He that dwells in the secret place of the most High shall abide under the shadow of the Almighty. I will say of the LORD, He is my refuge and my fortress: my God; in him will I trust. Surely he shall deliver you from the snare of the fowler, and from the noisome pestilence. He shall cover you with his feathers, and under his wings shall you trust: his truth shall be your shield and buckler. You shall not be afraid for the terror by night; nor for the arrow that flies by day; Nor for the pestilence that walks in darkness; nor for the destruction that waste at noonday. A thousand shall fall at your side, and ten thousand at your right hand; but it shall not come near you. Only with your eyes shall you behold and see the reward of the wicked. Because you have made the LORD,

which is my refuge, even the most High, your habitation; There shall no evil befall you, neither shall any plague come near your dwelling. For he shall give his angels charge over you, to keep you in all your ways. They shall bear you up in their hands, lest you dash your foot against a stone. You shall tread upon the lion and adder: the young lion and the dragon shall your trample under feet. Because he has set his love upon me, therefore will I deliver him: I will set him on high, because he has known my name. He shall call upon me, and I will answer him: I will be with him in trouble; I will deliver him, and honour him. With long life will I satisfy him, and show him my salvation." Psalm 91

20. In 2 Chronicles 16, Asa died in his sickness because he sought the physicians and not the Lord. While in Isaiah 38, Hezekiah lived because he sought the Lord and not the physicians.

21. God's Words always bring healing. As we read the Bible, healing comes to both our mind and body.

"Then they cry unto the LORD in their trouble, and he saves them out of their distresses. He sent his word, and healed them, and delivered them from their destructions." Psalm 107:19-20

"He heals the broken in heart (feelings, intellect), and binds up their wounds." Psalm 147:3

"My son, attend to my words; incline your ear unto my sayings. Let them not depart from your eyes; keep them in the midst of your heart. For they are life unto those that find them, and health to all their flesh." Proverbs 4:20-22

22. In Isaiah 53, the removal of our diseases is included in Christ's atonement, along with the removal of our sins. The word 'bare' implies substitution (suffering for), not sympathy (suffering with). If Christ has borne our sickness, why should we bare them?

"Surely he has borne our griefs, and carried our sorrows: yet we did esteem him stricken, smitten of God, and afflicted. But he was wounded for our transgressions, he was bruised for our iniquities: the chastisement of our peace was upon him; and with his stripes we are healed." Isaiah 53:4-5

23. In Matthew 8:16-17, Christ fulfilled Isaiah's words: *"healed all that were sick."*

"When evening came, they brought to Him many who were under the power of demons, and He drove out the spirits with a word and restored to health all who were sick. And thus He fulfilled what was spoken by the prophet Isaiah, He Himself took [in order to carry away] our weaknesses and infirmities and bore away our diseases." Mathew 8:16-17 AMP (see Isaiah 53:4)

24. In Job 2:7, sickness is revealed as coming directly from Satan. *"So went Satan forth from the presence of the LORD, and smote Job with sore boils from the sole of his foot unto his crown."* Job maintained steadfast faith as he cried out to God for deliverance, and he was healed. See Job 42:10, 12

25. In Luke 13:16 Christ declared that the infirm woman whom *"Satan has bound"* and that she ought to be loosed (set free). He cast out the *"spirit of infirmity,"* and she was healed. See Luke 13:11-16

26. In Matthew 12:22, a devil that possessed a man was the cause of his being both blind and dumb (inability to speak). When the evil spirit was cast out, he could both see and talk.

"Then was brought unto him one possessed with a devil, blind, and dumb: and he healed him, insomuch that the blind and dumb both spake and saw." Mathew 12:22

27. In Mark 9:17-27, a demon was the cause of a boy being deaf and dumb, and also the cause of his convulsions. When the demon was cast out, the boy was healed.

"And one of the multitude answered and said, Master, I have brought unto thee my son, which has a dumb spirit; And wheresoever he takes him, he teareth him: and he foams, and gnasheth with his teeth, and pines away: and I spoke to your disciples that they should cast him out; and they could not. He answers him,

and said, O faithless generation, how long shall I be with you? how long shall I suffer you? bring him unto me. And they brought him unto him: and when he saw him, straightway the spirit tare him; and he fell on the ground, and wallowed foaming. And he asked his father, How long is it ago since this came unto him? And he said, Of a child. And ofttimes it has cast him into the fire, and into the waters, to destroy him: but if your can do any thing, have compassion on us, and help us. Jesus said unto him, If you can believe, all things are possible to him that believes. And straightway the father of the child cried out, and said with tears, Lord, I believe; help my unbelief. When Jesus saw that the people came running together, he rebuked the foul spirit, saying unto him, you dumb and deaf spirit, I charge you, come out of him, and enter no more into him. And the spirit cried, and rent him sore, and came out of him: and he was as one dead; insomuch that many said, He is dead. But Jesus took him by the hand, and lifted him up; and he arose. Mark 9:17-27

28. In Acts 10:38, it is written: *"Jesus of Nazareth... who went about doing good, and healing all that were oppressed of the devil."* This scripture shows that sickness is Satan's oppression. And Jesus is the Healer!

29. In 1 John 3:8, we are told: *"The Son of God was manifested, that he might destroy the works of the devil."* Sickness

is part of Satan's works. Jesus, in His early ministry, always treated sin, diseases, and devils the same. They were all hateful in his sight. He rebuked them all. Jesus was sent from God the Father to destroy them all.

30. God does not want the works of the devil to continue in our physical bodies. He does not want cancer, a plague, a curse, *"the works of the devil"*, to exist in His own members.

"Know you not that your bodies are the members of Christ?" 1 Corinthians 6:15

31. Jesus said in Luke 9:56, *"The Son of man is not come to destroy men's lives, but to save them."* Sickness destroys; therefore, it is not from God. Jesus came to save us. In the original Greek translation of the Bible, the word save is the word "sozo", meaning 'to deliver us, to save and preserve us, to heal us, to give us life, to make us whole', but never to destroy us.

32. Jesus said in John 10:10, *"The thief (speaking of Satan) comes only to steal, and to kill, and to destroy: I am come that they might have life, and that they might have it more abundantly."*

Jesus said, *"I am the way, the truth, and THE LIFE: no man cometh unto the Father, but by me."* John 14:6

Satan is a killer; his diseases are the destroyers of life. His sicknesses are the thieves of happiness, health, money, time, and effort. Jesus Christ came to give us abundant life in our souls and in our bodies. Satan's work is to kill. Christ's work is to heal and give life.

33. All the old testament examples of God being the healer for Israel, apply to us today, and are given to us for an example.

> *"Now all these things happened unto them [Israel] for en-samples [examples or types]: and they are written for our admonition [attention], upon whom the ends of the world are come."* 1 Corinthians 10:11

Now with confidence, we can quote old testament examples of God being the healer of His people, and know they remain true today.

34. In 2 Corinthians 4:10-11, we are promised the life of Jesus in our mortal flesh.

> *"Always bearing about in the body the dying of the Lord Jesus, that the life also of Jesus might be made manifest in our body. For we which live are always delivered unto death for Jesus' sake, that the life also of Jesus might be made manifest in our mortal flesh."* 2 Corinthians 4:10-11

35. In Romans 8:11, we are taught that the Spirit's work is to quicken our mortal bodies in this life. The word 'quicken' in this scripture means to make alive, give life and vitalise. God wants to energize you.

> *"But if the Spirit of him that raised up Jesus from the dead dwell in you, he that raised up Christ from the dead shall also quicken your mortal bodies by his Spirit that dwells in you."* Romans 8:11

36. Satan is bad. God is good. Bad things come from Satan, so sickness is therefore from Satan. Good things come from God. Health is therefore from God. God can only give good things and never changes from this.

> *"Every good gift and every perfect gift is from above, and comes down from the Father of lights, with whom is no variableness, neither shadow of turning."* James 1:17

37. In Matthew 10:1, Mark 16:17, and Luke 10:19, all authority and power over all devils and diseases had been given to every disciple of Jesus Christ. Since Jesus said, *"If ye continue in my word, then are you my disciples indeed"* (John 8:31). These scriptures apply to you today, that is, if you continue in (act on) His Word.

38. In John 14:13-14, the right to pray and receive the answer is given to every believer. *"If you shall ask any thing in my name, I will do it."* This logically includes asking for healing, if we are sick. In Matthew 7:7-11, every one that asks receives. That promise is for you. It includes everyone who is sick.

> *"Ask, and it shall be given you; seek, and you shall find; knock, and it shall be opened unto you: For every one that asks receives; and he that seeks finds; and to him that knocks it shall be opened."* Mathew 7:7-8

39. In Luke 10:1,9,19, the ministry of healing was given to the seventy, who represent the future workers of the church - this includes Christians today.

Luke 10, Verse 1 "After these things the Lord appointed other seventy also, and sent them two and two before his face into every city and place, where he himself would come."

Verse 9 "And heal the sick that are therein, and say unto them, The kingdom of God is come near unto you."

Verse 19 "Behold, I give unto you power to tread on serpents and scorpions, and over all the power of the enemy: and nothing shall by any means hurt you."

40. In Mark 16:17, the ministry of healing was given to all of them that believe the Gospel, i.e., those who act on the gospel, or the practicers or doers of the Word (the Bible).

"And these signs shall follow them that believe; In my name shall they cast out devils; they shall speak with new tongues; They shall take up serpents; and if they drink any deadly thing, it shall not hurt them; they shall lay hands on the sick, and they shall recover." Mark 16:17-18

41. In James 5:14, the ministry of healing is committed to the elders of the church.

"Is any sick among you? let him call for the elders of the church; and let them pray over him, anointing him with oil in the name of the Lord:" James 5:14

42. In 1 Corinthians 12:9-10, healing is bestowed upon the whole church as one of its ministry gifts, that belongs to the church (that's us) until Jesus comes.

> *"To another faith by the same Spirit; to another the gifts of healing by the same Spirit; To another the working of miracles; to another prophecy; to another discerning of spirits; to another divers kinds of tongues; to another the interpretation of tongues:"* 1 Corinthians 12:9-10

43. We are told to pray for the sick and to know that our prayers will totally change the situation.

> *"Confess your faults one to another, and pray one for another, that you may be healed. The effectual fervent prayer of a righteous man avails much."* James 5:16

From this scripture, we can know that when we pray for the sick, our prayers accomplish many things and prevail in all situations. This includes praying for you own healing.

The Amplified Bible puts it this way:
> *"The earnest (heartfelt, continued) prayer of a righteous man makes tremendous power available [dynamic in its working]."* James 5:16 AMP

44. Jesus never commissioned anyone to preach the Gospel without commanding him to heal the sick. He said, *"Into whatsoever city he enter, ... heal the sick that are therein"* Luke 10:8,9.

That command still applies to the true ministry today.

45. Jesus said that He would continue His same works through believers while He is with the father. *"Truly, truly, I say unto you, He that believes on me, the works that I do shall he do also; and greater works than these shall he do also; because I go unto my father."* John 14:12. This certainly includes healing the sick. Jesus' earthly ministry included healing all those who were sick and oppressed, so our ministry should include these same works and also greater works.

46. In connection with the Lord's Supper, the cup is taken *"in remembrance"* of His blood which was shed for the remission of our sins. (1 Corinthians 11:25) The bread is eaten *"in remembrance"* of His body, on which were laid our diseases and the stripes by which *"We were healed."* 1 Corinthians 11:23-24; Is 53:5

47. Jesus said in Mark 7:13 that certain teachers were removing the effect and power of the Word of God because of their tradition. Man's ideas and theories have for centuries hindered the healing part of the Gospel from being proclaimed and acted upon as it was by the Early Church.

"Making the word of God of none effect through your tradition, which you have delivered: and many such like things do you." Mark 7:13

48. One tradition held by several people is that God wants some of His children to suffer sickness and that, therefore, many of the sick who are prayed for are not healed because

they think it is not God's will to heal them. When Jesus healed the demon possessed boy Mark 9, whom the disciples *"could not"* heal (v18), He proved that it is God's will to heal even those who fail to receive healing; furthermore, He assigned the failure of the disciples to cure the boy, not to God's will, but to the disciples' unbelief.

> *"Then came the disciples to Jesus apart, and said, Why could not we cast him out? And Jesus said unto them, Because of your unbelief: for truly I say unto you, If you have faith as a grain of mustard seed, you shall say unto this mountain, Remove hence to yonder place; and it shall remove; and nothing shall be impossible unto you."* Matthew 17:19-20

49. The failure of many to be healed today when prayed for is never because it is not God's will to heal them. Remember He is Jehovah Rapha - the Lord that heals.

50. If sickness is the will of God, then every physician would be the law-breaker, every trained nurse a defier of the Almighty, and every hospital a house of rebellion instead of a house of mercy!

51. Faith is a key to receiving your healing. To have 'faith' means to believe what the Bible promises, without doubting or wavering, to visualize, act and speak what the Bible says. Faith will bring into existence those things that you hope for. We can see from the following scriptures that faith was the key to these healings:

"And He said to her, Daughter, your faith (your trust and confidence in Me, springing from faith in God) has restored you to health. Go in (into) peace and be continually healed and freed from your [distressing bodily] disease. Mark 5:34 AMP

"And the prayer of faith shall save the sick" James 5:15

"Therefore I say unto you, What things soever you desire, when you pray, believe that you receive them (have faith), and you shall have them." Mark 11:24

52. Since Jesus came to do the Father's will, the fact that He *"healed them all"* is proof that it is God's will that all be healed.

"All they that had any sick with divers diseases brought them unto him; and he laid his hands on every one of them, and healed them." Luke 4:40

53. If it is not God's will for all to be healed, how did *"every-one"* in the multitudes obtain from Jesus what was not God's will for some of them to receive? The Gospels say several times, *"He healed them all."* Mathew 4:24, 12:15, Luke 4:40, 6:19.

54. If it is not God's will for all to be healed, why do the Scriptures state: *"With his stripes we are healed and by whose stripes you were healed?"* (Is.53:5;1 Pet.2:24) How could "we" and "you" be declared healed, if it is God's will for some of us to be sick?

_____

55. The bible teaches that healing is His children's bread. In other words, healing is part of the food to sustain them and keep them strong.

> *"And, behold, a woman of Canaan came out of the same coasts, and cried unto him, saying, Have mercy on me, O Lord, thou Son of David; my daughter is grievously vexed with a devil. But he answered her not a word. And his disciples came and besought him, saying, Send her away; for she cries after us. But he answered and said, I am not sent but unto the lost sheep of the house of Israel. Then came she and worshipped him, saying, Lord, help me. But he answered and said, It is not right to take the children's bread, and to cast it to dogs. And she said, Truth, Lord: yet the dogs eat of the crumbs which fall from their masters' table. Then Jesus answered and said unto her, O woman, great is your faith: be it unto you even as you will. And her daughter was made whole from that very hour."* Matthew 15:22-28

56. Jesus never refused those who sought His healing. Repeatedly, the Gospels tell us that He healed them all. Christ the Healer has never changed!

> *"Jesus Christ the same yesterday, and to day, and for ever."* Hebrews 13:8

57. Only one person in the entire Bible ever asked for healing by saying, *"If it be Your will"*....That was the poor leper

to whom Jesus immediately responded, *"I will; be you clean (healed)"* Mark 1:40-41

58. You are healed before you see the sickness or disease leave your body.

> *"Who his own self bare our sins in his own body on the tree, that we, being dead to sins, should live unto righteousness: by whose stripes YOU WERE HEALED."* 1 Peter 2:24

The price for your healing was paid for when Jesus went to the cross. It was accomplished then, and now by faith, you can receive what was already paid for.

In Matthew 8:17, we read, "And thus He fulfilled what was spoken by the prophet Isaiah, He Himself took [in order to carry away] our weaknesses and infirmities and bore away our diseases." Jesus is not taking away our diseases, he TOOK them.

59. A traditional thought is that we can glorify God more by being patient in our sickness, than by being healed. If sickness glorifies God more than healing, then any attempt to get well by natural or divine means would be an effort to rob God of the glory that we should want Him to receive.

60. If sickness glorifies God, then we should rather be sick than well. No one who has experienced sickness wants to remain sick. You cannot serve, worship and glorify God unhindered if you are sick.

Sickness does not glorify God, otherwise Jesus robbed His Father of all the glory that He possibly could, by healing everyone (Luke 4:40), and the Holy Spirit continued doing the same throughout the Acts of the Apostles.

61. In 1 Corinthians 6:20, Paul says, "*You are bought with a price: therefore glorify God in your body, and in your spirit, which are God's.*" Our bodies and our spirits are bought with a price. We are to glorify God in both. We do not glorify God in our "spirit" by remaining in sin. We do not glorify God in our "body" by remaining sick.

62. John 11:4 is used to prove that sickness glorifies God, but God was not glorified in this case until Lazarus was raised up from the dead. The result of this was that many of the Jews believed what Jesus said and did.

> "*Then many of the Jews which came to Mary, and had seen the things which Jesus did, believed on him.*"
> John 11:45

63. Another tradition is that while God heals some, it is not His will to heal all. But Jesus, Who came to do the Father's will, did "*heal them all*". If this is the case, why did Jesus bear "our" sicknesses, "our" pains, and "our" diseases? If God wanted some of His children to suffer, then Jesus relieved us from bearing something which God wanted us to bear. But since Jesus came to do the "*will of the Father*" and since He "*hath borne our diseases,*" it must be God's will for all to be well.

64. If it is not God's will for all to be healed, this would mean that the Bible is only true for some people and does not apply to all. A conclusion like that would also mean that faith does not come by hearing the Word of God alone, but by getting a special revelation that God has favoured you and wills to heal you. God would then be showing favour to some people and not to others. The Bible clearly says this is not the case:

"For there is no respect (partiality, favouritism) of persons with God." Romans 2:11

65. If God's promises to heal are not for all, then we could not know what God's will is by reading His Word alone. This would then mean, we would have to pray until He speaks directly to us about each case in particular. We could not consider God's Word as directed to us personally, but would have to close our Bible and pray for a direct revelation from God to know if it is His will to heal each case. That would be absurd and lead to total confusion! Rest assured God's Word is for all who believe, and that includes you.

66. God's Word is His will. God's promises reveal His will. When we read of what He promises to do, we then know what His will is.

67. Since it is written, *"Faith comes by hearing...the word of God"* (Romans 10:17), then the best way to build faith in your heart and life for healing that would be to listen to the part of God's Word, which promises you healing.

68. Faith for spiritual healing (salvation) comes by hearing the Gospel: He bore our sins. Faith for physical healing comes by hearing the Gospel: He bore our sicknesses.

"Who (speaking of Jesus) his own self BARE OUR SINS in his own body on the tree, that we, being dead to sins, should live unto righteousness: by whose stripes you were healed." 1 Peter 2:24

"That it might be fulfilled which was spoken by Esaias (Hebrew for Elijah) the prophet, saying, Himself took our infirmities, and BARE OUR SICKNESSES." Matthew 8:17

69. We are to preach the Gospel to every creature. The word Gospel literally means 'good news or good message.' This good news includes that *"He bore our sins"* and that *"He bore our sicknesses."*

"And he said unto them, Go ye into all the world, and preach the gospel (good news/message) to every creature." Mark 16:15

70. In John 14:12-14, Jesus emphasised His promise by repeating it twice, *"If you shall ask anything in my name, I will do it."* He did not exclude healing from this promise. *"Anything"* includes healing. This promise is for all.

If healing is not for all, Jesus should have qualified His promise in Mark 11:24 accordingly, and said, *"What things soever you desire (except healing) when you pray, believe that you receive them, and you shall have them."* But He did not. Healing, therefore, is included in the *"what things soever."* This promise is made to you!

71. If it is not God's will to heal all, the promise Jesus made in John 15:7 would not be reliable.

"If you abide in me, and my words abide in you, you shall ask what you will, and it shall be done unto you." John 15:7

By having the Word of God abide in you, you can know without any doubt that you can ask for healing *"and it shall be done unto you."*

72. In James 5:14-15 we read: *"Is any sick among you? let him call for elders of the church; and let them pray over him, anointing him with oil in the name of the Lord: and the prayer of faith shall save the sick, and the Lord shall raise him up."* This promise is for all, including you, if you are sick.

73. Jesus Christ was *"made to be sin for us"* (2 Corinthians 5:21). When He was made to be sin, He exchanged our sin for His righteousness (right standing with God).

"For he has made him to be sin for us, who knew no sin; that we might be made the righteousness of God in him." 2 Corinthians 5:21

The price Jesus paid exchanged our sinful nature for His righteousness, so to did this price pay for our sickness and infirmities.

Jesus *"bare our sins"* (1 Peter 2:24), and was *"made a curse for us"* (Galatians 3:13), when *"He bare our sicknesses."* (Matt: 8:17)

---

74. Paul tells us that God would have us *"prepared unto every good work"* (2 Timothy 2:21), *"thoroughly furnished unto all good works"* (2 Timothy 3:17), *"that we may abound to every good work"* (2 Corinthians 9:8). A sick man cannot measure up to these scriptures. These conditions would be impossible if healing is not for all. Either healing is not for all, or these scriptures do not apply to all.

75. Bodily healing in the New Testament was called a *"mercy"*, and it was God's mercy, which always moved Him to heal all the sick. His promise is that He is *"plenteous in mercy unto all that call upon Him"* (Psalm 86:5). That includes you today.

76. The correct translation of Isaiah 53:4 is: *"Surely (or certainly) He has borne our sicknesses, and carried our pains."* To prove that our sicknesses were carried away by Jesus Christ, just like our sins were carried away, the same Hebrew verb for *"borne"* and *"carried"* is used to describe both. (See verse 11-12)

77. If God today has abandoned healing in answer to prayer (divine healing) in favour of healing only by medical science, as modern theology speculates, that would mean that He requires us to use a less successful method during a *"better"* dispensation (time period defined by major Biblical events). He healed them all then, but today many diseases are incurable by medical science. This would mean that people were better off before Jesus came to the earth, which is clearly not the case.

78. Since Christ bare our sins, how many people does God want to forgive? Answer: *"Whosoever believes."* (John 3:16) Since Christ bares our sicknesses, how many people does God want to heal? Answer: *"He healed them all."* (Luke 6:19)

79. Another tradition is that if we are righteous, we should expect sickness as a part of our life. They quote the scripture: *"Many are the afflictions of the righteous"* (Psalm 34:19), but this does not mean *"sickness"* as some would have us believe. It means trials, hardships, persecutions, temptations, etc.; but never sickness or physical disabilities.

80. It would be a contradiction to say, *"Christ has borne our sicknesses, and with His stripes we are healed,"* but then add, *"Many are the sicknesses of the righteous, which He requires us to bear."*

81. To prove this tradition that was mentioned in the previous point, people sometimes quote, *"But the God of all grace, who hath called us unto his eternal glory by Christ Jesus, after that ye have suffered a while, make you perfect, establish, strengthen, and settle you"* (1 Peter 5:10). This 'suffering' does not refer to suffering sickness, but to the many ways in which God's people have so often had to suffer for their testimony. (See Acts 5:41; 2 Corinthians 12).

82. Another tradition is that we are not to expect healing for certain 'afflictions.' They quote the scripture, *"Is any among you afflicted? Let him pray"* (James 5:13). This again does not refer to sickness, but to the same things pointed out previously in number 78.

83. Another tradition is that God chastises His children with sickness. They quote the scripture in Hebrews 12:6-8, a part of which says, *"Whom the Lord loves he chasteneth (corrects)."* This is true. God does chasten those He loves, but it does not say that He makes them sick. The word "chasten"

here means to "instruct", train, discipline, teach, or educate, like a teacher "instructs" his pupil, or like a father "trains and teaches" his child. God "chastens" us by His Holy Spirit and by His Word (the Bible).

84. The most common tradition is the worn out statement: 'The age of miracles is past.' For this to be true, there would have to be a total absence of miracles. Even one miracle would prove that the age of miracles is not past.

85. When a teacher "instructs" his student, he may employ various means of discipline, but never sickness. When a father "trains" his child, he chastens (corrects) by different means, but never by imposing a physical disease upon him. For our heavenly Father to "chasten" us does not require that He lay a disease upon us. Our diseases were laid upon Jesus. God could not require that we bear, as punishment, what Jesus has substitutionally borne for us. Christ's sacrifice freed us forever from the curse of sin and disease which He bore for us.

86. If the age of miracles is past, no one could be born again because the new birth is the greatest miracle in the world.

87. If the age of miracles is past, as some claim, that would mean that all the technical evidence produced in hundreds of laboratories of the world, concerning innumerable cases of miraculous healings, is false and that God's promises to do such things are not for today.

88. Healing is a good gift from God. In Acts 10:38 we read, *"How God anointed Jesus of Nazareth with the Holy Ghost and with power: who went about DOING GOOD AND HEALING all that were oppressed of the devil; for God was with him."*

We also read in Matthew 7:11, *"If you then, being evil, know how to give good gifts unto your children, how much more shall your Father which is in heaven give good things to them that ask him?"*

Now we see that healing is good, and that God shall give good gifts to His children.

89. When Jesus sent His disciples to preach the Gospel, He told them: *"These (supernatural) signs shall follow them that believe"* (Mark 17:16). This was for every creature, for all nations, until the end of the world. The end of the world has not yet come, so the age of miracles has not passed. Jesus' Commission has never been withdrawn or annulled.

90. The age of miracles is not past because the Miracle-Worker has never changed: *"Jesus Christ the same yesterday, and to day, and forever."* Hebrew 13:8

91. Anyone who claims that the age of miracles is past denies the need, the privileges, and the benefits of prayer. For God to hear and answer prayer, whether the petition is for a postage stamp or for the healing of a cripple, is a miracle. If prayer brings an answer, that answer is a miracle. If there are no miracles, there is no reason for faith. If there are no miracles, prayer is a mockery, and only ignorance would cause a man to either pray or expect an answer.

God cannot answer prayer without a miracle. If we pray at all, we should expect that prayer to be answered. If that prayer is answered, God has done it; and if God has answered prayer,

He has performed something supernatural. That is a miracle. To deny miracles today is to mock prayer today.

92. Christ's promise for the soul-that it shall be saved-is in the Great Commission and is for all. His promise for the body-that it shall recover - is in the Great Commission and is for all. To deny that one part of the Great Commission is for today is to deny that the other part is for today. As long as the Great Commission is in effect, sinners can be healed spiritually, and sick people can be healed physically by believing the Gospel. Multiple thousands of sincere people all over the world are receiving the benefits of both physical and spiritual healing through their simple faith in God's promises.

93. Christ bore your sins so that you may be forgiven. Eternal life is yours. Claim this blessing and confess it by faith; God will make it good in your life.

94. Christ bore your diseases so that you may be healed. Divine health is yours. Claim this blessing and confess it by faith; God will manifest it in your body.

95. Like all of Christ's redemptive gifts, healing must be received by simple faith alone without natural means and, upon being received, must be consecrated for Christ's service and glory alone.

96. Since Romans 8:32 is true today, God is as willing to heal His worshippers as He is to forgive His enemies. That is to say, if when you were a sinner, God was willing to forgive you, now that you are His child, He is willing to heal you. If He was merciful enough to forgive you when you were His enemy,

He is merciful enough to heal you now that you are His worshipper and His child.

97. A person must accept God's promises as true and believe he is forgiven before he can experience the joy of spiritual healing. The sick person must accept God's promise as true and believe he is healed before he can experience the joy of physical healing.

98. *"As many (sinners) as received him...were born...of God"* (John 1:12,13) *"As many (sick) as touched him were made whole."* (Mark 6:56) When we declare it is always God's will to heal, the question is immediately raised: *"How then could we ever die?"* Well God's Word says *"You take away their breath, they die, and return to their dust"* (Psalm 104:29). In Job 5:26, we read: *"You shall come to your grave in a full age, like as a shock of corn comes in his season."*

99. God the Father has prepared a table of provision and abundance for us in the midst of our enemies. Sickness and disease are clearly one of the tools that Satan uses against us. But God has prepared a way out of sickness and disease for His children.

"You prepare a table before me in the presence of my enemies." Psalm 23:5

100. For us to come to our full age and for God to take away our breath does not require the aid of cancer or any other disease. God's will for the death of His children is that, after we have lived a fruitful life and fulfilled the number of our days. We simply stops breathing and falls asleep in Christ. Only to

awaken on the other side and live with Him forever. *"So shall we ever be with the Lord"* (1 Thessalonians 4:17). Indeed, this is the blessed hope of the righteous.

> *"Because he has set his love upon me", God says, "therefore will I deliver him: I will set him on high, because he has known my name. He shall call upon me, and I will answer him: I will be with him in trouble; I will deliver him, and honour him. With long life will I satisfy him, and show him my salvation"* Psalm 91:14-16

101. The most important fact about healing is this, God is love. God not only has love, God is love. *"He that loves not knows not God; for GOD IS LOVE."* 1 John 4:8

> *"Love endures long and is patient and kind; love never is envious nor boils over with jealousy, is not boastful or vainglorious, does not display itself haughtily. It is not conceited (arrogant and inflated with pride); it is not rude (unmannerly) and does not act unbecomingly. Love (God's love in us) does not insist on its own rights or its own way, for it is not self-seeking; it is not touchy or fretful or resentful; it takes no account of the evil done to it [it pays no attention to a suffered wrong]. It does not rejoice at injustice and unrighteousness, but rejoices when right and truth prevail. Love bears up under anything and everything that comes, is ever ready to believe*

the best of every person, its hopes are fadeless under all circumstances, and it endures everything [without weakening]. Love never fails [never fades out or becomes obsolete or comes to an end]. As for prophecy (the gift of interpreting the divine will and purpose), it will be fulfilled and pass away; as for tongues, they will be destroyed and cease; as for knowledge, it will pass away [it will lose its value and be superseded by truth]. 1 Corinthians 13:4-8 AMP

Knowing that God is love, and that He loves you, you must know that God wants you to be healthy, prosperous and live a long life. Always be a blessing, as you are blessed with 'The Blessing of Abraham' through Jesus Christ. *"And if you are Christ's, then you are Abraham's seed, and heirs according to the promise."* Galatians 3:29. God promised Abraham that through Him, all the families of the earth would be blessed. Sickness is not a blessing, it is a curse. Jesus Christ came to set us free from the curse of the law. That we might receive the promise of the Spirit by faith, that is 'The Blessing of Abraham', and live forever in relationship with Him. A loving relationship with God, through our Lord Jesus Christ.

Prayerfully read these facts over and over. Meditate upon them and allow the Holy Spirit to birth the faith and the revelation of them down in your spirit. Jesus Christ paid the full price for you to be healed and enjoy life. Constantly speak these truths over your body and circumstances. There is life in the power of your words.

Chapter Seven

HEALED OF CORONAVIRUS

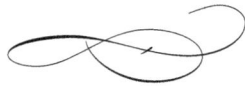

Before I close this book, I would like to share a further two testimonies that I have witnessed firsthand through my humble prayers. I give all the glory to God for these healing miracles.

Recently, at the height of the Covid-19 pandemic outbreak in England, I received a phone call from a member of my church congregation.

Jim had called in, requesting urgent prayer for his son, Corey. Corey is a schoolteacher in London. He had been struck down by the Corona Virus. He had collapsed at home with extreme breathing difficulties and was coughing up blood. His wife called the ambulance, but due to the hundreds of other emergencies, waited four hours, and still, no ambulance had arrived.

After further phone calls by his wife to the emergency hospital department, she was instructed to call an Uber to take Corey to hospital as they couldn't give a time when an ambulance would come due to an unprecedented overload on their emergency resources.

The Uber came and rushed Corey along with his wife to the emergency department. Corey describes the scene that he was to enter as horrendous. The emergency ward was packed to capacity and over-flowing. People were passing out, gasping for air and in agony with extreme breathing difficulties. He waited for a while, and eventually, a health emergency worker said to him "you will have to go home as we have nowhere to put you, we are over-run, and there are people in a worse state than you".

His wife called another Uber and helped her extremely sick husband to the car and eventually to his home. Corey collapsed in bed and was gravely ill from the virus. From her London home, his wife called his parents, Jim and Laraine in Brisbane, Australia and told them of the dire condition their son was in and how he had been sent home with no medication or anything.

Jim and Laraine immediately called me, and I entered a prayer of agreement with them for their son's deliverance and miracle healing. I took authority over the spirit of infirmity, rebuking it in the name of Jesus and commanding it to come out of their son's body. I commanded the Corona Virus to die and leave his body in Jesus mighty name. I prayed that the Holy Spirit would quicken and give life to his mortal flesh freeing up his lungs and bronchial breathing passages.

Jim and Laraine were later to learn that from that moment of prayer their son Corey began to recover and get well. Corey has made a full recovery from the Corona Virus and is now back teaching.

Corey learned that a co-worker that had suffered the same conditions as he did, later died from them.

Jim and Laraine, their son Corey and his wife, give all the glory to God for his miraculous recovery, and they say it was the prayer that saved his life.

Chapter Eight

NINE STEPS TO DIVINE HEALING

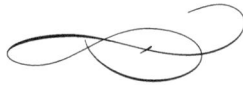

1. Remember, sickness is from Satan.

Be settled in your own heart and mind that sickness is not from God - it originates from Satan.

2. Know it is God's will to heal you.

Be settled in your own heart and mind that it is the will of God to heal you. Jesus came to do the will of God (John 6:38) and never once did He refuse healing to those who came in faith. Do not pray *"....if it be Your will."* To doubt God's will is to doubt God's promises. What God has promised, He is willing and able to do. Moreover, as sickness is the "oppression of the devil", it is obviously God's will to set you free. (Acts 10:38)

3. Cast aside all fear!

Jesus said, *"Fear not; believe only and (you) shall be made whole."* (Luke 8:50) The Bible frequently exhorts us to fear not. Fear undermines our faith. Kenneth Copeland says,

"Fear tolerated is faith contaminated." We must deal with our fears first, then exercise our faith in the promises of God.

4. Forgive everybody.

Mark 11:25-26 shows that unforgiveness is very definitely a hindrance to receiving answers to our prayers - *"And when ye stand praying, forgive, if ye have ought against any; that your Father also which is in heaven may forgive you your trespasses. But if ye do not forgive, neither will your Father which is in heaven forgive your trespasses."* Take the initiative and sincerely forgive all who have sinned against you or have done you wrong or harm. Don't hold a grudge or have bitterness towards another person. Allow God's love to remove it from your life. Now allow God's forgiveness and love to flow through you to all others.

5. Have a positive attitude of mind!

Where there is true faith in a person's heart, it is shown in a positive, cheerful and confident attitude. Learn to think, speak and act positively. There is tremendous power in positive believing. Jesus said, *"If you can believe, all things are possible to him that believe"* Mark 9:23.

In your imagination, your mind's eye, see yourself as God sees you, healed!

6. Base your faith on God's promises.

Read many times over and over the scriptures given in these notes and any others that are of special meaning to you. Learn to base your faith, not on your feelings nor your circumstances, but on the infallible promise of God and His Word.

7. Release your faith, in the Name of Jesus

We all have a measure of faith (Romans 12:3). The only difference is that some use their faith and others don't. Faith must be released to be effective. Sooner or later, there comes a time when your faith is turned loose - perhaps as you read this teaching, or when hands are laid on you in the Name of Jesus, or some other time when you definitely release your faith and put it into action.

> Acts 3:16 states, *"And his name through faith in his name has made this man strong, whom you see and know: yes, the faith which is by him has given him this perfect soundness in the presence of you all."*

Notice it was the **Name of Jesus** and faith in that name that got the man healed.

8. Resist the symptoms.

Recognise that sickness originated from the devil, and God is the author of your healing. Learn to resist the devil, and as the Bible says, *"he will flee from you."* James 4:7. We do not deny the symptoms for they are real enough, but we deny their right and power to remain any longer in our bodies in the face of God's mighty promises on which we now believe, and base our faith, standing steadfast, knowing that, *"what God has promised, He is also willing and able to perform."* (Romans 4:21).

Now do something you could not do! Remember, **faith is an act.** (James 1:22).

9.   Praise and thank God continually.

Praise is joyously thanking God for something He has done or promised to do. So then in regard to your healing, thank God continually by saying that *"by the stripes that Jesus bore for me at the Cross of Calvary, I was healed."* (Taken from 1 Peter 2:24).

In 1 Corinthians 15:57, it says that *"praise or thanks to God gives you victory through our Lord Jesus Christ."*

Remember, *"Death and life are in the power of the tongue"* (Proverbs 18:21). So watch the words of your mouth. Only say what God says about your healing and future and trust in Him to bring it to pass. Thank Him, that in the mighty **Name of Jesus**, you are healed!

God's Promise to You

Because he has set his love upon me, therefore will I deliver him: I will set him on high, because he has known my name. He shall call upon me, and I will answer him: I will be with him in trouble; I will deliver him, and honour him. With long life will I satisfy him, and show him my salvation. Psalm 91:14-16

NINE STEPS TO DIVINE HEALING REVISION

Your homework for this lesson is to go over and over these nine points, and study the scriptures.

The following are some scriptures from God's word for you to meditate on and use to build your faith for healing. Remember, Romans 10:17, *"So then faith comes by hearing, and hearing by the word of God."*

"And you shall know the truth, and the truth shall make you free." John 8:32.

"Jesus Christ the same yesterday, and today, and forever" Hebrews 13:8.

"Every good gift and every perfect gift is from above, and comes down from the Father of lights, with whom is no variableness, neither shadow of turning." James 1:17.

"Surely he hath borne our griefs, and carried our sorrows: yet we did esteem him stricken, smitten of God, and afflicted. But he was wounded for our transgressions, he was bruised for our iniquities: the punishment of our peace was upon him; and with his stripes we are healed." Isaiah 53:4-5.

"And you shall serve the LORD your God, and he shall bless your bread, and your water; and I will take sickness away from the midst of you." Exodus 23:25.

"And said, If thou wilt diligently hearken to the voice of the LORD thy God, and wilt do that which is right in his sight..... for I am the LORD that heals you." Exodus 15:26.

Boldly declare, in the Name of Jesus that God is your Healer!

"Beloved, I wish above all things that you may prosper and be in health, even as your soul prospers." 3 John 1:2.

Joyously thank and praise Him, that you are healed and prospering in your day!

CHAPTER NINE

SET FREE BY THE LAW OF LIFE

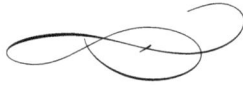

The Law of the Spirit of Life

This new kingdom is a spiritual kingdom, but just because salvation is basically a spiritual rebirth does not mean that it has no effect on our bodies, minds, or everyday living. It can and should have a great impact on every part of our lives.

In every age and culture, there are certain rules and laws that govern the actions of the inhabitants of that area. It is the same in spiritual life. There are laws for those in Satan's kingdom, and there are laws for those in God's kingdom. The new birth gives us a new law. ***"FOR THE LAW OF THE SPIRIT OF LIFE IN CHRIST JESUS*** *hath made me free from the law of sin and death"* (Romans 8:2).

The law of life includes love, joy, peace, happiness, prosperity, abundance, health, contentment, and blessings. These provisions are made for the Christian in the New Covenant. We must enforce them in our lives. As we enforce them, God will back us. He always enforces His Word, which is true and never changes. His Word is law and forever settled in heaven.

Forgiveness of All Our Sins

The day we make Jesus our Lord and Saviour we are forgiven of all our sins, in fact, we were legally forgiven when Jesus gave His life as a ransom for us. But we do not experience that forgiveness until we receive it by faith.

Although a person may have committed many sins, the chief sin of the unsaved is **NOT BELIEVING ON CHRIST** (John 16:9). When a person gets that straightened out, the root of the problem is solved. The blood of Christ cleanses the heart the moment a person believes and confesses Him as Saviour. Thus all past sins are remitted or taken away by the powerful cleansing work of His blood (1 John 1:7). *"... We have redemption through His blood, the forgiveness of sins, according to the riches of His grace."* (Ephesians 1:7).

Here is a simple prayer you can pray in order to be born again:

Father, I come before you in the precious name of Jesus.
Lord, I have made mistakes in my life.
Father, I acknowledge that I have sinned.
I see in Your Word it says that Jesus died for my sins. Please forgive me of all of my sins and mistakes against you that I have committed, or any other person that I may have wronged.
I forgive all those who have sinned against me or

wronged me in any way.
Father, I repent right now of my sins.
Father, I thank You that You sent Jesus, who came in the flesh and died for me, taking my sins on the cross, shedding His blood for me. Thank you, I am now clean from my sins, through the shed blood of Jesus Christ. Thank you that on the third day You rose Jesus again from the dead. Jesus now sits at Your right hand in all power and glory, as King and Lord of all.

Jesus, please come into my life, my heart, right now by the Person and power of the Holy Spirit, and make me born again.
Jesus, I receive You now as my Lord and my Saviour. Amen.

Welcome to God's Family

If you prayed this simple prayer, you can know, according to God's Word that you are saved. You are now born again and have become a Christian, a follower of Christ. You must stand on His Word, not your feelings, emotions, or anything else. It is God's Word that guarantees your salvation, which includes spiritual, mental and physical healing.

Assurance of Salvation

"And this is the record that God has given to us eternal life, and this life is in His Son. HE THAT

HAS THE SON HAS LIFE, *and he that has not the Son of God has not life. These things have I written unto you that believe on the name of the Son of God;* **THAT YOU MAY KNOW** *that ye have eternal life, and that ye may* **BELIEVE ON THE NAME** *of the Son of God."* (1 John 5: 11-13).

The Resurrection and the Life

Jesus said, "I am the Resurrection and the Life. He that believes in Me, though he were dead, yet shall he live. And whosoever lives and believes in Me shall never die." (John 11:25-26).

Isn't that wonderful? I encourage all who read this, to embrace this truth from the Word of God. Today, receive Jesus Christ as your personal Lord, Saviour, healer of your body and restorer of your soul. Your name will then be found in the Lord's Book of Life. (Revelation 3:5, 20:15 & Luke 10:20).

Chapter Ten

PUNCTURED LUNG HEALED

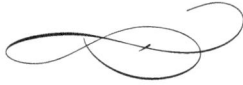

A few years ago, a member of my church car had broken down in our church car park. Rob, a member of our congregation at the time, had a friend who was a mechanic. I called Rob to see if he could come with his mechanic friend and have a look at the car. Rob said, "No worries Ps Shaun, I'll bring my mechanic mate, and we will come over and have a look at the car".

When Rob arrived at the church property, his friend, the mechanic started to work on the car, and Rob stood there holding his side, and it was very obvious to me that he was in pain, had difficulty breathing and with his movement.

I asked Rob, "What's the matter with you?" to which he replied, "I did something very silly, Ps Shaun. I rounded up my horses the other day into the coral, and I climbed up on the fence to climb over one horse to sit on another horse to ride it out. The first horse I climbed over bucked and I went flying in the air and landed on the top of the coral wooden fence post."

Rob went on to explain how that he was in so much pain that he went to his doctor who subsequently sent him for an x-ray, which showed he had a broken rib that had punctured his left lung, which had then filled up over one third with blood and fluid.

His doctor told him that he would schedule surgery and send him in for an operation to have the blood and fluid drained from the lung. The doctor wanted to keep Rob in over-night, immobilizing him in bed so that they could perform the operation as soon as possible.

Rob told the Doctor, "No, let me go home, and I promise you I will just sit in my armchair, watch TV and not move." The doctor reluctantly agreed to Rob's request because Rob was so adamant and persistent that he was going home. They couldn't operate for a day or two anyway, and so Rob promised his doctor he would go home, sit still and not move while he waited for the call. He promised his doctor that if he grew any worse or had any greater difficulty breathing, he would come straight back in, in an ambulance.

I said to Rob, "What are you doing here?!" He said, "Well I was sitting at home waiting for the call from the hospital when you called Ps Shaun, so I decided to come here instead".

I had my son, Nathanael with me at the time so I said, "Come on Nathanael lets pray a prayer of faith for a healing miracle for Rob right now. You lay your hands on one side of Rob's body, and I will lay my hands on the other side."

So standing there, under the gum trees in the church car park, we gently laid hands on Rob's chest and side. I commanded the spirit of infirmity to be loosed and leave Rob's body. I commanded the rib to heal, the lung to heal, the fluid to go and the pain to cease, in the mighty name of Jesus, declaring that by the stripes that Jesus bore Rob is healed. I took authority, spoke to the lungs in Jesus name and commanded and demanded they line up with the word and be made whole.

The following day Rob went back to his doctor, who said to him I'm just going to take another x-ray before surgery to assess the situation before we operate.

Rob sat in the waiting room after his x-ray waiting for the results before they wheeled him into the operating room for the procedure.

The doctor came in with the new x-rays, put them on the board and said "Rob, take a look at these. I want to ask you a question, where did the blood go?"

Rob told me he said to the doctor "How do I know where the blood went? You're the doctor, you tell me". To which the doctor replied, that's the problem; I can't, because I have no idea where the blood went. Not only that, take a look at the lung that was damaged, it's completely healed, and it is in better condition than the right lung, which wasn't punctured.

Rob came to church the following week and held up the x-rays of his lungs before and after showing the improved condition of the one that had been miraculously healed by prayer given in the name of Jesus.

———

I give God all the glory for his goodness and his wonderful works to the children of men.

CHAPTER ELEVEN

THE WAYS OF GOD

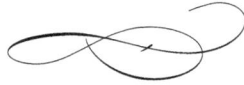

"He made known his ways unto Moses, his acts unto the children of Israel." Psalm 103:7

God uses different ways to heal. As we have stated earlier in this book, all healing comes from God. Every promise of God is received into our life by faith.

God Rewards Faith

It states in Hebrews 11:6, *"But without faith it is impossible to please him: for he that comes to God must believe that he is, and that he is a rewarder of them that diligently seek him."*

What this verse really means, is that it takes faith to receive God's promises into our life. These promises have been provided for us by Jesus through the price He paid on the cross. Like our salvation is received by faith, in the same way, healing must be received by faith.

Kenneth Hagin, that great faith teacher (I highly recommend you read all Hagin's work on faith), said, "Faith begins where the will of God is known." We have to know it is God's will to heal us, just as much as we know it is God's will to save us.

> In Romans 10:17 it states, *"So then faith comes by hearing, and hearing by the word of God."*

We are going to get the faith that we need to receive our healing by meditating God's Word.

> Joshua 1:8 says, *"This book of the law shall not depart out of your mouth; but you shall meditate therein day and night, that you may observe to do according to all that is written therein: for then you shall make your way prosperous, and then you shall have good success."*

The meaning of the word 'meditate' in this scripture is not just listening and studying. It also implies a speaking, muttering over and over. We could say a confession of the Word until a mental image is formed in our mind, of the desired result. This being the victory or healing you desire that has been provided for you by Christ. See yourself well!

See and Speak Yourself Well

Faith will come as you read God's Word, hearing it in your mind, but it will come faster if you read God's Word aloud with boldness and passion.

Hear yourself read and speak the Word of God! Listen to yourself speaking and confessing His promises boldly.

Say what the Word says! Speak to the mountain, the problem, telling it to leave. Then expect this to happen even before you see it or feel it.

Faith sees the unseen. Faith sees with the spiritual eye what the natural eye cannot yet see. See it done with your spiritual eyes, the eyes of faith!

> In Mark 11:23 - 24, *"For truly I say unto you, That whosoever shall say unto this mountain, be removed, and be cast into the sea; and shall not doubt in his heart, but shall believe that those things which he says shall come to pass; he shall have whatsoever he says. Therefore I say unto you, what things soever you desire, when you pray, believe (expect) that you receive them, and you shall have them."*

We must believe and expect that we will receive it before we actually have it, in order to receive it. This is the God kind of faith; Faith that calls the things that aren't as though they already existed.

> Romans 4:17 says, *"(As it is written, I have made you a father of many nations,) before him whom he believed, even God, who makes alive the dead, and calls those things which be not as though they were."*

Abraham grew strong in faith, giving glory to God, and he was fully persuaded that what God had promised, He was able to also perform (Romans 4:20-21).

Abraham had an attitude of gratitude, was a worshipper and a lover of God. He expressed this to God by giving Him glory and praising Him.

Four Things God Desires

God desires four things from us. He wants us to love Him with all our hearts. He wants us to love each other. He wants us to believe His Word. He wants us to do His Word (be doers of the Word).

In Matthew 9:29 it says, *"Then touched he their eyes, saying, according to your faith be it unto you."*

Everyone is going to receive everything they get from God, according to their faith. All the blessings of God come to us according to our faith.

The Apostle Paul said in Philippians 3:10, "That I may know him, and the power of his resurrection, and the fellowship of his sufferings, being made conformable unto his death;"

The more we get to know God, the more we will understand the power of His resurrection. Jesus accomplished so much for us at Calvary when He died and then rose from the dead. Healing is part of the redemption that was purchased for us by Jesus Christ.

In Romans 5:2 it says, *"By whom also we have access by faith into this grace wherein we stand, and rejoice in hope of the glory of God."*

We access God's grace by faith. In this book, we have covered some of the different methods that God uses to heal, but the result is always the same. God wants us whole, healed and prospering in life.

In the Old Testament, God revealed Himself to His people by His redemptive names; here we see 'I am the Lord that heals you' is Jehovah Rapha. The word 'Jehovah' in Hebrew, means that God is the self-existent One who is forever, always bringing Himself into existence. He is the Life-Giver, Creator, He who brings things to pass, the performer of His Promises. 'Rapha' in the Hebrew means to heal. To be completely healed, become fresh (new). Rapha also means, physician. It means to take care of and to be repaired or healed. So we could say that God is the Healer.

God, who is always bringing His promises to pass in our lives, because it is His divine will, promises that you are healed, repaired, renewed and made whole.

Remember, Jesus came to earth to do the will of His Father. He went to the cross and paid the price for your healing, as well as your sins. God wants you well! His desire is for you to enjoy your life and all of the blessings He has provided for us in Jesus, and His Kingdom.

Be Led by the Spirit

God will, by His Holy Spirit, lead you into all truth. The Holy Spirit will teach you and birth understanding of these things to your spirit as you pray to the Father in Jesus name.

Paul said in Ephesians 1:16-18 says, *"Cease not to give thanks for you, making mention of you in my prayers; That the God of our Lord Jesus Christ, the Father of glory, may give unto you the spirit of wisdom and revelation in the knowledge of him: The eyes of your understanding being enlightened; that you may know what is the hope of his calling, and what the riches of the glory of his inheritance in the saints,"*

God uses different ways to heal or to manifest the healing in our bodies. In chapters 3, 4 and 5 of this book, we have covered some of the different ways that healing is administered and received. But it is God that works the miracle in us as He wills.

We have covered anointing with oil, the laying on of hands, casting out of devils, the command faith, receiving through being a child of Abraham, through Christ and the blessing of Abraham. We have looked at confessing and receiving your miracle by faith.

As you study the Word of God, through His Word you will find many and varied ways in which healing was administered and received. Even in the testimonies I have included, healing came to the people I prayed for, in different ways.

Another way that I have seen God do amazing miracles is through the anointing of handkerchiefs, prayer cloths and other personal items. I remember, back in the '90s, when on several occasions I travelled to Czechoslovakia with Dr. Steve Ryder, seeing this miracle work in action.

Steve ministered healing to the thousands of people that were coming to hear about Jesus. Great healing miracles were taking place. Steve would minister through the laying on of hands. As he was doing this, people, due to the sheer numbers wanting prayer and the long prayer lines, started to pass items of clothing to the front. They wanted Steve Ryder to touch these garments and pray over them.

Steve instructed us to get a table to put the clothes and personal items on. I will never forget the mound of clothing; jackets, jumpers, scarfs, shoes, handkerchiefs and blankets that piled high, on this table. Steve would then go over and in front of everyone, pray over and lay hands on the pile, imparting the anointing in the name of Jesus. The clothes would then be passed back to the owners. I was amazed as I watched this work, over and over. Everything just seemed to go back to the right people. As people put those clothes back on, miraculous healings would take place. Over the following days, many people would come and testify of how they and other family members were healed, from those pieces of clothing when they were placed on their bodies.

Miracles of Healing in India

Learning from Steve Ryder, this was one of the methods I used in the great healing campaigns that I conducted in India.

Up to two hundred thousand plus people would gather in a single meeting. In one of these meetings, our ministry purchased twenty thousand prayer cloths, printing them with our logo to be handed out at the meeting. I explained to the people the scripture from the book of Acts, the same scripture that Steve had used in Czechoslovakia.

> Acts 19:11-12 says, *"And God wrought special miracles by the hands of Paul: So that from his body were brought unto the sick handkerchiefs or aprons, and the diseases departed from them, and the evil spirits went out of them."*

I then proceeded to lay hands on the prayer cloths, praying over them and believing to impart the anointing. These would then be passed out to the people to take home to their sick family members, who were not able to come at the time, to receive the laying on of hands.

We received many testimonies of great and miraculous healings. One testimony I remember, was from a doctor who had a blind daughter. The doctor attended our meeting. He came forward for prayer and healing and at the same time, asked if he could have a prayer cloth, that I had prayed over. I took the cloth and laid hands on it, imparting the anointing, in the mighty name of Jesus. The doctor took that prayer cloth home and that night laid it on the eyes of his blind daughter, as she slept in her bed. Praise God, the next day, his daughter woke up crying that she could see! All the glory goes to Jesus!

We still regularly receive handkerchiefs and prayer cloths in the post. People write in and they ask me to pray over these items and anoint them in the name of Jesus. Many people have been healed through this and other methods, by which we have released our faith for their miracles, as outlined in this book.

It is faith in the name of Jesus that causes the healing miracle to manifest. The cloth, oil or the laying on of hands is just a point of contact, where people can release their faith to receive.

In 1 Corinthians 12: 4-11, it talks about the different gifts and how they work and are administered differently. But it is the same Lord that works them all, through us His people.

> "Now there are diversities of gifts, but the same Spirit. And there are differences of administrations, but the same Lord. And there are diversities of operations, but it is the same God which works all in all. But the manifestation of the Spirit is given to every person to profit everyone. For to one is given by the Spirit the word of wisdom; to another the word of knowledge by the same Spirit; To another faith by the same Spirit; to another the gifts of healing by the same Spirit; To another the working of miracles; to another prophecy; to another discerning of spirits; to another divers kinds of tongues; to another the interpretation of tongues: But all these works that one and the self-same Spirit, dividing to every person severally as he will." 1 Corinthians 12:4-11

As we read the above scripture, we can see that the gifts of the Holy Spirit operate in different ways at different times, through different people. When we become born again, we don't become like robots. God still uses our different personalities. Even though we are one as a body, we are still individuals'. As we grow in the Spirit, The Holy Spirit will flow through us in different ways at different times.

We can also see, from the above scripture, that there are different gifts and different administrations of those gifts. The gift of the working of miracles is different from the gift of healing.

Let me share a couple of powerful healing miracles that I have personally witnessed through my humble prayers and commands of faith, that I have released in the name of Jesus.

Many years ago, during one of my trips to India, I ministered in a small village called Vatsavai in Kammam. After preaching on the power of the cross and the blood, I gave an altar call for salvation, followed by one for healing. People came from all over that village and lined up to receive healing prayers, through the laying on of hands. I will never forget an elderly grandmother, who brought her baby grand-daughter to the front for prayer. The baby's mother had died giving birth and now the baby was being raised by her grandma. The baby could sit up, but her head flopped over to one side when the grandmother let it go. Even though the child was now at an age where she should be easily able to support her own head weight, she wasn't able to do so.

It was scary to watch as the grandmother sat the baby on the stage and her head fell down to her chest or shoulder. Through the interpreter, the grandmother expressed that the baby had no muscles or strength in her neck to support the head weight. I did not know if this baby was paralysed, had a broken neck or was simply born with deformed or no neck or shoulder muscles.

I laid hands on the baby and prayed for her, there was no change, so I handed her back to her grandmother. She moved to the back of the line, where she re-joined it and waited her turn to reach the front again for further prayer. I prayed for the baby again, cast out every spirit of weakness and commanded the neck to be healed in Jesus name! Nothing happened. I handed the baby back to the grandmother. She moved to the back of the line and lined up again. This process went on all night. Nothing happened. There was no change to the little girl.

The next night, after my faith message, it came time for the prayer line again. This same grandmother, with the same baby stood and waited for prayer. I prayed, nothing happened and she went to the back and lined up again. That grandmother was so persistent in prayer that she persisted doing this every night for four nights. In front of everybody, I prayed for that little girl dozens of times each night. On the fourth night, the last night of our meetings in that village, the grandmother came for prayer with the little girl once again. By now, everyone was angry with her. Many people were receiving miracles through the laying on of hands. Everyone thought that this lady was selfish because she lined up so many times. I admired her persistency. I admired her perseverance.

I will never forget, on that last night when that grandmother pushed her way through the crowds of people wanting prayer and shoved the baby girl in my hands. I took the grandmother and in front of everybody passed the baby back to her. I laid hands on the little girl in that grandmother's arms. The power of God pulsed through my hands and into that little body. Next minute the grandmother was crying and shouting that the little girl's head was healed! I took the little baby and sat her on the stage that night in front of everyone, including my team from Australia.

Every person had tears in their eyes. I was crying too. The little girl was looking around from side to side, sitting up with a perfectly straight neck and head. Another amazing part of this miracle, is when that surge of God's Holy Ghost anointing power, went out of my hand and into the baby's body. It went through the baby and unbeknownst to me, the grandmother had a huge lump on her forearm, like a tumour. It was giving her a lot of pain. She never once asked for prayer for herself, just for that child. But the power of God went through that baby, healing her neck and into the grandmother's forearm. The tumorous lump and pain disappeared. The grandmother, who was holding the child with the perfectly healed neck, stood on the stage that night giving glory to God for His wonderful healing power and His goodness. We all rejoiced with her at God's magnificence and goodness, for both her and her granddaughter's healing.

God Moves the Same in Africa

In Malawi Africa, I recall another powerful healing testimony. I was ministering in Geoffrey Matoga's church in the city of

Blantyre. Pastor Geoffrey was a mathematics professor at the local university, whom God had called into the ministry. While I was a part of a large healing campaign where thousands were being healed and set free by the power of God, I had the pleasure of meeting Geoff, who was one of the supporting churches and pastors of the campaign.

Pastor Geoffrey invited me to come on Sunday and speak at his church. After I had finished preaching, I called for people to come to the front who needed prayer for healing. One brother made his way to the front. As he came, I noticed he was wearing a leg brace down one entire leg and had two crutches under his arms. When he stood before me, I looked down at his feet and I could see that one leg was extremely shorter than the other. Under the leg with the steel brace, the man had his shoe built up with a block of wood, approximately four inches or ten centimeters thick. I can honestly say that this was one of the biggest differences in a person's leg length that I had seen. Usually, people come for prayer and they may have one leg a centimeter or up to an inch shorter than the other.

This problem had caused the man to have extreme lower back pain and disability all his life. There he stood before the whole crowd of people in the church that day. I said to the people, I have just declared "Jesus, as the Healer. Now let's see what Jesus can do." I reached out to lay hands on that brother that day, and as I did, I commanded the spirit of infirmity to come out of him. I then commanded his leg to grow out and be the same as the other!

I will never forget that day! Before my hands touched his head and while I was speaking the commands of faith, in the name of Jesus, the brother fell backwards to the ground. I had a couple of men there as ushers/catchers, as is my practice when I am praying on prayer lines. These brothers caught him and assisted his fall to the ground. I instructed them to let him lay there for a while under God's wonderful healing presence and anointing.

I then said to the church, "Let's lift the man up and see what God has done." Well, to everyone's utter amazement, the short leg had grown out four inches (10cm) to be the same length as the other leg. Upon standing him up, I had to get four bibles from the audience, which I placed under the good leg to match the height of the leg with the brace and wooden block. As you can imagine, everyone was praising God and after this everyone wanted to receive prayers of faith. The man went to the restrooms and removed his brace and the wooden blocks and then returned to the meeting, showing everyone his legs as he walked and stood at the front, that were now both the same length!

Forgiveness

Give Satan No Place

One of the most powerful triggers that I have used to cause the great miracle power of God to flow is forgiveness. When I have stood before the crowds of people that have come to hear the good news and receive prayer for healing, I always teach on the power of forgiveness.

It says in Mark 11:24-25, *"Therefore I say unto you, what things so ever you desire, when you pray,*

*believe that you receive them, and you shall have
them. And when you stand praying, forgive, if you
have anything against anyone: that your Father also
which is in heaven may forgive you your mistakes
and sins. But if you do not forgive, neither will your
Father which is in heaven forgive your sins, mistakes
and wrongdoings."*

From this verse of scripture, we can see the importance that
the Father, God in heaven, places upon forgiveness. The bible tells us in Hebrews 4:16, *"To come boldly to the Throne
of Grace that we may receive mercy and find grace (favour) to
help in our time of need."* In Genesis 8:22, we read about the
law of seedtime and harvest. In life, we reap what we sow! If
we want to reap forgiveness from our heavenly Father from all
of our wrongs, we must first sow forgiveness to those that have
wronged us.

I like to say that unforgiveness is a violation of grace. Forgiveness is a powerful divine and Godly grace that has its roots
in love. Remember, God is love. God, Jesus, instructs us in
His Word to love everyone.

The Force of Forgiveness

Forgiveness is a deliberate decision to release feelings of
resentment or vengeance toward a person or group who has
harmed you, regardless of whether they actually deserve your
forgiveness. The word forgiveness, amongst other things,
means "to let it go". We can see from the above verses of
scripture that if we want our prayers answered, if we want to
receive our breakthrough, healing or miracle, we must forgive.

When we hold unforgiveness in our heart towards others, it doesn't hurt them but rather hurts and can cause a root or roots of bitterness to spring up within our emotions and our being. This then can lead to all kinds of sickness and ailments, as our body is not functioning as God designed it. A merry heart, the Word says, does us good like a medicine. It's God's medicine to our soul and body. It causes and fosters a ground for faith to grow. The Word calls this, *"Faith that works by love."* Galatians 5:6.

During a four day crusade, I would dedicate each night to a different message. I would be led by the Spirit in the precise message for those people, but I would base my messages on God's goodness (prosperity), God's love, God's healing and salvation and God's forgiveness. I would ask everyone to join me in a sincere prayer, where we would pray out loud and forgive everyone who has ever sinned against us or wronged us, in any way. I would then get them all to ask God to forgive them and lead them in a prayer to be born again and led by the Spirit, through their lives.

As God then directed or impressed me, I would call out words of knowledge, as led by the Spirit of God. During this time, many great healing miracles would manifest all over the crowd. I would do this, and then ask people to come to the front and testify of the good things that God had done in their bodies. After the testimonies, I would then proceed to lay hands on and minister healing to everyone that came and joined the prayer lines.

Healing by Word Knowledge

One testimony that comes to mind is from a man who is a pastor and still keeps in contact with me. From the pulpit, I said, "There is a man here, I believe you are in ministry, you have travelled a long way to be here. You have just received word that your son has been struck down with paralysis. You are very worried about your son. The Lord tells me to tell you, that He is being healed as we speak and you will receive word that he is fine. So you can have faith that God is in control and looking after and healing your son while you are here."

Later after the meeting, I met this man. His name is John Victor. He was a pastor who had travelled a long way, many miles by train to my meeting to hear me speak and receive prayer for his ministry. This was before the days of mobile phones. Before the meeting, he had called home on a land-line and received the news of his son's condition, just like the word of knowledge I gave. His son was gravely ill, having been struck down by some kind of virus/flu. He was unable to walk and very sick. I use this illustration to teach how healing can manifest through a word of knowledge. His son received healing that night.

After the meeting, Pastor John Victor called home and received the good news of his son's miracle. Today, Pastor John works as one of our pastors in Potnuru, India. His son is grown up, married and now has children of his own. To this day, Pastor John rejoices for the miracle healing power of God, that I spoke forth that evening by a word of knowledge regarding his son.

The bible says that we overcome the evil one by the blood of Jesus and the word of our testimony (Revelations 12:11).

We need to testify of the great things God has done in our lives by His goodness and grace. In Psalm 107 it says, "Oh that men would praise the Lord for His goodness and His wonderful works to the children of men."

When we testify of God's goodness, we take the focus off of our problems and we put the focus on God's goodness and promises in His Word. In 1 Corinthians 13:13 it says, "And now abide faith, hope, love, these three; but the greatest of these is love."

"Faith comes by hearing and hearing by the Word of God" (Romans 10:17).

When we hear a testimony, it inspires us to reach out in faith to the love of God. God in His great love paid a great price through the sacrifice of His son Jesus at the cross, for us to receive salvation, healing, deliverance and prosperity. God loves you and wants you well!

Praying in Tongues – Strengthening the Inner Man

As we have listed in this book, there are many ways through which this healing can manifest. The Lord wants to fill us with His Spirit and give us the ability to pray in tongues. When we pray in tongues, we energize ourselves. Praying in tongues is a supernatural ability that God gives, that enables the believer to water their faith by releasing and speaking a supernatural audible language of the Spirit. Your faith is strengthened and you are refreshed in your spirit and soul, as you enter into the rest of God by praying in tongues.

I have found that through spending hours praying in tongues before the great healing campaigns I have conducted throughout the world, that I have experienced an increase in faith that has led to the release of the other eight gifts of the Spirit. These have operated at different times as the Spirit has led. God has used me to release, gifts of healing, working of miracles, discerning of spirits, prophecy and even the gift of faith. I explain the gift of faith as a self-energizing belief. It is like, you have built your faith to one level, but when the gift of faith manifests in you, you can believe for the impossible to become possible. I honestly believe that as we push into God and are faithful to study His Word ("Study to show yourself approved unto God, a workman that needs not to be ashamed, rightly dividing the word of truth" 2 Timothy 2:15.), there is no limit to how much we can grow and achieve in Him. All things are possible to those who believe (Mark 9:23). God wants you well!

Miracles in India

I have been so blessed in my life to see so many healing miracles over the years. The following are the kind of the testimonies that Raj collected of healings that took place in our meetings in India, in different towns and localities. He has many more, but there are too many to include. I include these to inspire you to reach out in faith, with a hope (confident and favourable) to receive all of God's best for you and the promises contained in His Word, based on His great love for you.

Healing Testimonies from Raj Kiran

Fifteen-year-old Ms Rani had suffered from schizophrenia for four years. She suffered many hysterical bouts. Nobody was able to cure her. Then Pastor Shaun prayed over her and she changed. The demonic possession had left and she is now leading a normal life!

Ms Kumari, 30, has three children. Her husband was a casual worker at construction sites. Two years ago, during the construction of a building, a boulder fell on to him. He was crushed under the impact. Most of his major bones were fractured. It took him almost two years to recover, yet his sternum bone didn't heal and as a result, he was bedridden. The economic consequences on his family were enormous. They starved for most of the time.

Last December, friends helped him to the "World Harvest Ministries" meetings. At the time, he was a Hindu. After being prayed for by Pastor Shaun, he was a changed man. He returned home totally transformed. He gained faith in the Lord and His miracle healing power. Slowly his sternum bone began healing and now he is totally healed.

Venkata Rao, 65, was working in a sugar factory as a casual labourer. He is married with four children. Over a year ago he fell into a crushing machine which broke many of his bones.

It has taken more than a year for the bones to heal, but still he remained immobile. He went from place to place in search of a miracle cure. Finally, he was brought to the World Harvest Ministries meetings. Pastor Shaun prayed for his healing.

Now he is able to limp with the help of crutches and can use his hands for washing and eating. He is so overjoyed that he wants to become a Pastor. He sends his blessings to all the team at WHM.

Twenty-two year old Mrs Kumari, married a truck driver five years ago. They have a daughter aged 1 ½. One rainy night her husband's truck crashed into a giant tree and turned over. Passers-by got him out of the truck and rushed him to hospital. He was in a coma and was declared a hopeless case. Mrs Kumari heard about WHM's meetings. Accompanied by her mother, she attended the meetings and prayed for her husband, and on the third day after the prayers, her husband came out of the coma and regained consciousness. Within a week he was discharged from hospital and is now back truck driving. Praise God!

Ms Radha, 28, married Krishna Rao, 13 years ago and has four children. Her husband became an alcoholic. He drank and drank and stopped working. It went on for more than eight years. He started beating her and the children. On many occasions she ran to her parents' home along with her children, unable to bear his drunken brawls. He would not take any advice from friends and family to change his life. Then one close friend brought the couple to the World Harvest Ministries meetings. After Pastor Shaun prayed over him, he changed. He now shuns alcohol. He goes to work and his family is happy and united, thanks to the restoration and healing power of the Lord. Mrs Radha sends her thanks to the World Harvest Ministries team.

Rajendra Prasad, 40, is working for a government office. "I can't be silent about what I saw at your miracle crusades," he said. "I saw God's presence around Pastor Shaun during the crusades. I saw a bright glory light around him." Before the crusade, I was a Hindu and suffered from high blood pressure. It was 210/170. Even after long term treatment, it stayed high. Doctors told me I was developing kidney trouble. Now I am free of all diseases. I received healing when you stretched forth your hands and prayed. Now my blood pressure is 160/90."

"Over the years," Raj says, "I have collected these and hundreds of other testimonies from the healing and blessing prayers of Dr Shaun Marler. Huge uncountable miracles happened over a 25 year journey. I have eye-witnessed so many miracles of healing and deliverance, along with unexplainable manifestations of God's glory. Blind eyes have opened, people born deaf have started to hear. The mute have spoken. Stroke victims have regained the use of their arms and limbs again. People have testified of many other ailments and maladies healed through Dr Shaun's prayers. I have even had people write in and send photos of leprosy, before and after, that has left their body.

I am glad that I am still alive to share my personal firsthand experience of God's Spirit and power working through and in Dr Shaun. In each and every rally, both the large outdoor campaigns as well as indoor halls and conference centres, where the name of Jesus was proclaimed, the power of God manifested. People received healing and great joy and wonderment were in the meetings. Dr Shaun Marler would always give all the glory to God and tell all present, that Jesus loves them."

Photos from Dr Shaun Marler's Healing Campaigns

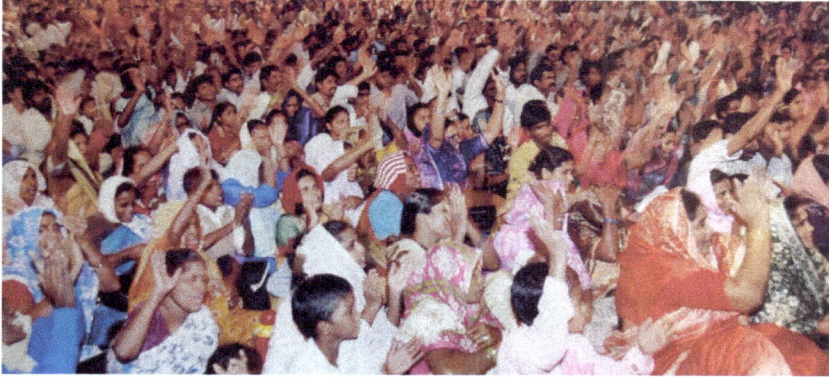

Crowds of people raising their hands to receive Christ as Saviour.

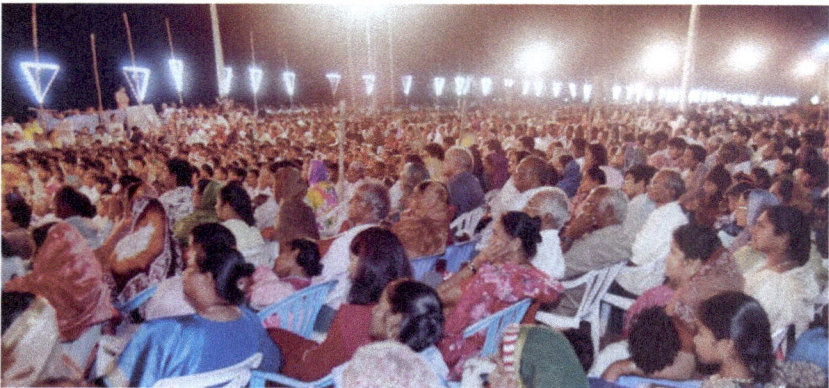

Tens of thousands sit and listen as Dr Shaun shares on God's great love.

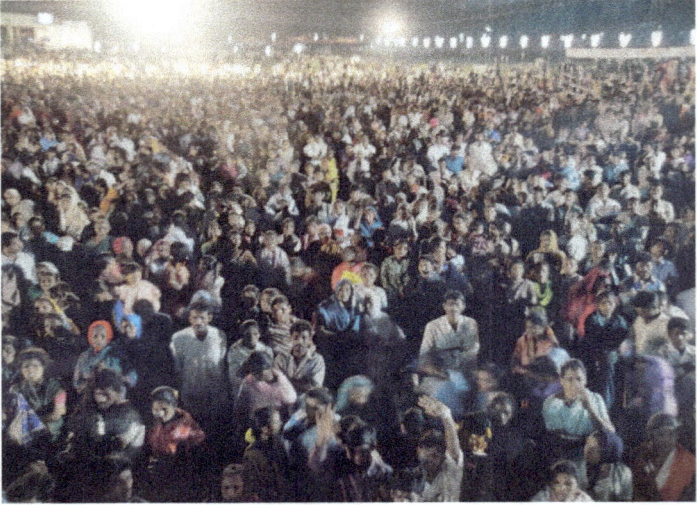

Kakinada, India Healing Rally ,where over 200,000 gathered to hear Dr Shaun Marler preach the Word and demonstrate God's healing power.

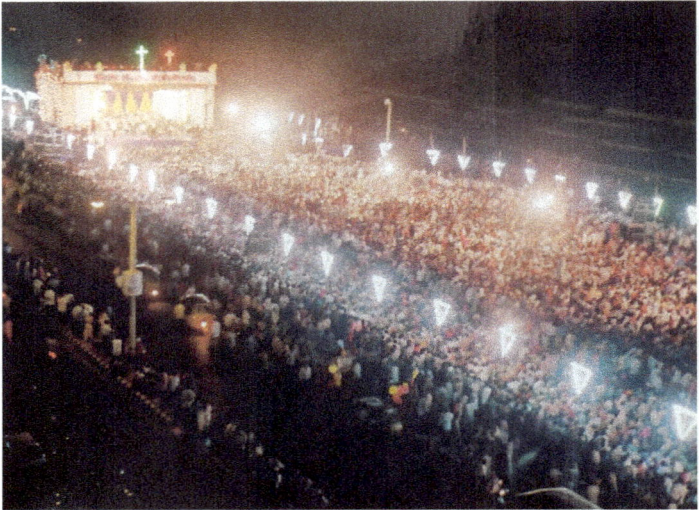

Visakhapatnam, India 'Festival of Praise and Healing', where more than 100,000 people attended.

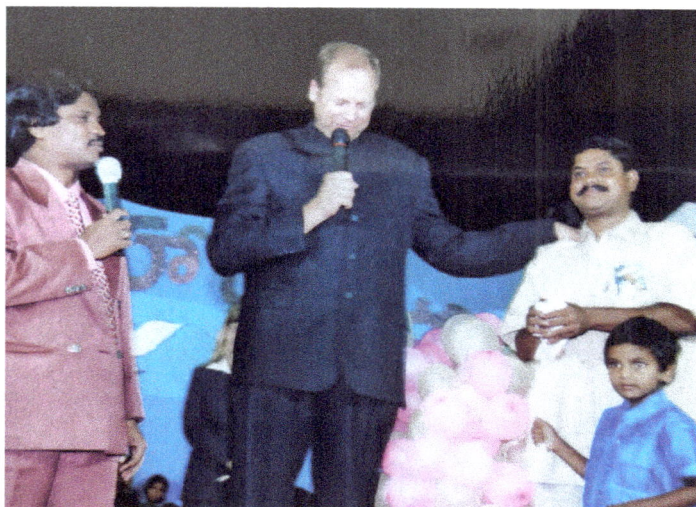

Dr Shaun praying for Raj Kiran with his interpreter Dr Suvartharaju.

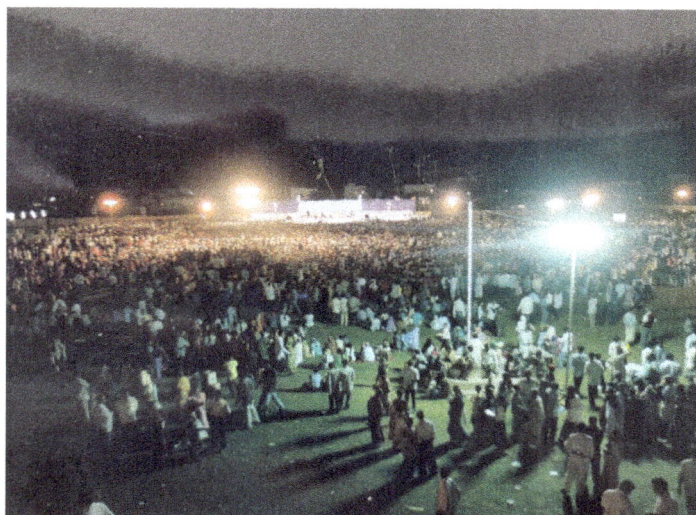

Overhead shot looking towards the platform of another great healing campaign in India ,from where Dr Shaun delivered a life-changing message and thousands received healing miracles.

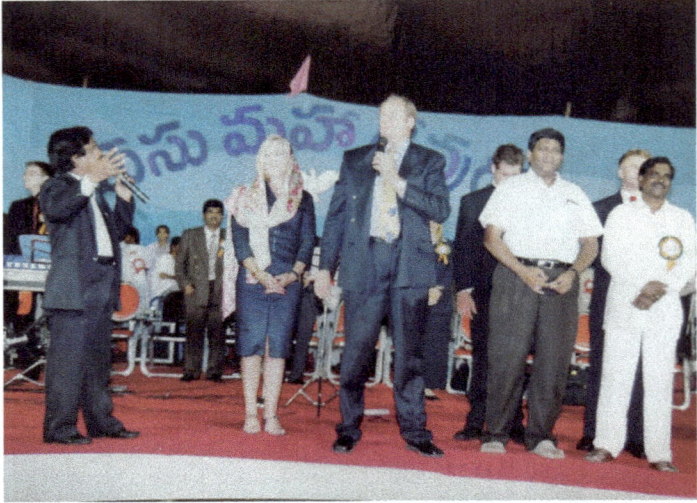

*Dr Shaun and Kerrie Marler praying for God's blessings
and prosperity on the nation of India.*

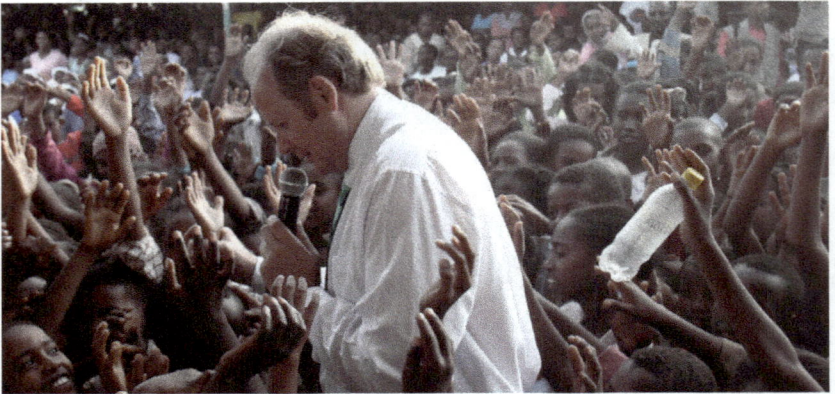

*Dr Shaun laying hands and praying for healing at one of the
'Festival of Healing and Praise' meetings in Ethiopia, Africa.*

CHAPTER TWELVE

LAUGHTER

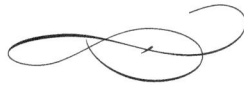

Never forget, that Jesus not only went to the cross to die and pay the price for your sins, but He also took your diseases and sicknesses in His body, becoming a curse in order that you may be healed. The price for your healing has been paid in full!

Many years ago I read a book titled, 'He Who Laughs, Lasts and Lasts and Lasts'.

In Proverbs it says, **"A merry heart does us good like a medicine."** So don't forget to laugh.

Laughter is an ability placed in us by God when we were created. He placed this ability within us, enabling us to express our enjoyment through life. As we laugh, we harness its powerful benefits. God says, *"It will do us good, like a medicine."* Proverbs 17:22. Scientists have discovered that a good laugh triggers healthy, physical and emotional changes in the body.

Laughter actually strengthens your immune system, boosts mood, diminishes pain and helps protect you from the damaging effects of stress. Laughter releases endorphins and healing chemicals. These hormones and chemicals decrease stress hormones while increasing immune cells and infection fighting antibodies. This improves your resistance to disease.

Laughter inspires hope and helps us to release anger and unforgiveness towards others. Destructive attitudes and emotions that Satan uses to keep us bound and broken in life.

God has placed in us, this incredible ability to laugh in the face of all opposition. When we choose to laugh and rejoice, we actually release healing chemicals within our bodies that protect the heart by improving the function of blood flow vessels, increasing blood flow. Once again, this decreases pain, relieves anxiety and strengthens resilience.

Laughter helps prevent heart disease.

Laughter is attractive. It enhances teamwork, attracts others to us and helps diffuse conflicts.

In Zephaniah 3:17 it declares, *"God rejoices over us with joy."* Jesus rejoiced as he approached the cross. Because laughter helps shift perspective, from the problem to the answer. It will get you out of your head and into the answer, which is the word of God. It will help keep you focused on the prize, the victory you have in Christ.

A good hearty laugh relieves physical tension and stress, leaving your muscles relaxed for up to forty-five minutes after.

Joy and laughter reconnects us with God and others. It improves our emotional health, strengthening our relationships and adding years to our life.

We are truly fearfully and wonderfully made (Psalm 139:14).

John G. Lake.

The following is John G. Lake's consecration to the Lord. John G. Lake was a great healing apostle and evangelist from the last century. His life and writings have inspired me and encouraged me to reach for God's best. You will be inspired by reading testimonies of great and miraculous healings from this man's ministry. For further books and information on Apostle John G. Lake, please refer to the footnotes in this book.

Dr John G. Lake 1920

"First commit your body and soul and spirit in entire, hundredfold consecration to God forever. Do not be satisfied with sins forgiven. Press on, press in, let God have you and fill you, until consciously He dwells, lives, abides in every cell of your blood, of your bone and your brain, until your soul (psychic) (mind), indwelt by Him, thinks His thoughts, speaks His word, until your spirit assimilates God, and God's Spirit assimilates you, until your humanity and His divinity are merged into His eternal Deity. Thus BODY, SOUL and SPIRIT are God's forever and forever. Amen. THAT is the POWER OF DIVINE HEALING. Behold I give you power...over all the power of the enemy: and nothing shall by any means hurt you (Luke 10:19)."

A final word from the author...

God wants you well. Jeremiah 29:11 says, *"For I know the thoughts that I think toward you, saith the Lord, thoughts of peace, and not of evil, to give you a hope and a future."*

Now thanks be unto God, who always causes you to triumph. (2 Corinthians 2:14).

We have established in this book that Satan is the source of sickness. Jesus Christ is the source of our miraculous healing. He came *"That He might destroy the works of the devil"* 1 John 3:8.

Jesus said in John 10:10, *"I have come that you might have life and that you may have it more abundantly."*

Your best is still to come!

"For better is the end of a thing, then the beginning thereof" (Ecclesiastes 7:8).

If you have received your healing through speaking and applying the teaching of this little book. Please write in and let us know. We would love to hear the wonderful testimonies of what God has done!

Email: general@whm.org.au

Because he has set his love upon me, therefore will I deliver him: I will set him on high, because he has known my name.

He shall call upon me, and I will answer him: I will be with him in trouble; I will deliver him, and honour him.

With long life will I satisfy him, and show him my salvation.

PSALM 91 - 14-16

YOU ARE COMPLETE IN CHRIST!

FOOTNOTES

In presenting these 101 Divine Healing Facts, we are indebted to the resourceful writings of T.L. Osborne author of 'Healing the Sick', and F.F. Bosworth, from which several of the thoughts expressed have been gleaned and expanded upon.

F.F. Bosworth's faith literature has brought healing within the grasp of many thousands who could not have recovered without knowing the truths, which it contains. By reading his book, 'Christ the Healer', you can get in just a few hours what took Rev. Bosworth thirty years of hard work in the healing ministry all over the U.S.A. and Canada to learn. I urge every Christian, pastor, teacher, and evangelist to obtain a copy of this masterpiece in faith building, and to read it repeatedly.

I have personally listened to and read the teachings of T.L. Osborne for over thirty-five years. I highly recommend you acquire and read his faith building, inspiring and encouraging material.

Other Recommending Reading

"He Who Laughs, Lasts, Lasts and Lasts" by Roy H. Hicks.
"Healed of Cancer" by Dodie Osteen.
"Healing Promises" by Kenneth and Gloria Copeland.
'Adventures in God' by John G. Lake.
*To read Kerrie Marler's full testimony of her healing. Please obtain a copy of her book, "Miracles Never Cease" Coming to an online bookstore soon.

N.B. Scripture from the KJV bible has been modernized by the author for reading and understanding purposes. E.g. *He that hath the Son hath life'*, has been changed to, *'He that has the Son has life'*.

ABOUT THE AUTHOR

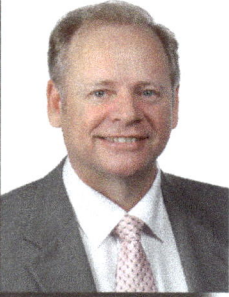

Dr Shaun Marler is the Senior Pastor and co-founder with his wife Kerrie of World Harvest Ministries, an international organisation based in Queensland, Australia, World Harvest Ministries is committed to carrying out the Great Commission of Jesus our Lord. Taking the healing word to the nations and feeding the hungry, visiting prisoners, clothing the naked, visiting the widows and orphans in their affliction, and preaching the Good News to the poor.

World Harvest Ministries currently has programs in Australia, Africa and India, where the poor and destitute are given free medical treatment, orphan homes where children are fed, accommodated and educated, a ministry to widows who have been abandoned by society and a program to feed people with leprosy.

A portion of the proceeds of the sale of this book goes towards this valuable work, which is making a huge difference in the lives of others!

Also by Dr. Shaun Marler

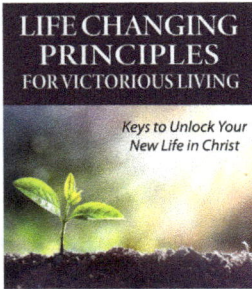

Life Changing Principles For Victorious Living.
Foreword by noted authors, Jerry Savelle, Col Stringer and Jim Kilbler.
Life Changing Principles for Victorious Living is a must read! You will find keys to unlock your life in Christ.

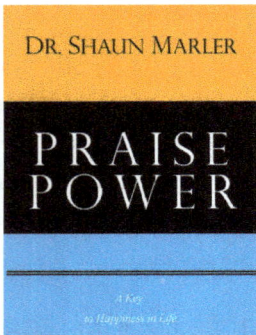

Praise Power
Foreword by Dr Reg Klimionok
Everything in your life is subject to change. God's will for your life is that it changes for the better. How do you get there? Through praise in the Word, because praise is the verbal expression of Faith and Faith is the language of Heaven.

These books and other titles are available on Amazon as well as other online bookstores around the world!

Partnership

Help Pastor Shaun to help others, by becoming a Harvest partner in this great work of spreading the gospel and loving others.

Please email general@whm.org.au and become a World Harvest partner today!

For other information and a complete list of products, or to find out how you can partner with the ministry of Dr Shaun Marler and World Harvest Ministries, contact:

P.O. Box 90 Bald Hills 4036
Phone: +61 7 3261 4555
(9am – 4:30pm EST Aust)
Web: whm.org.au
Email: general@whm.org.au
Facebook: www.facebook.com/worldharvestmin
Facebook: www.facebook.com/ShaunMarlerWHM

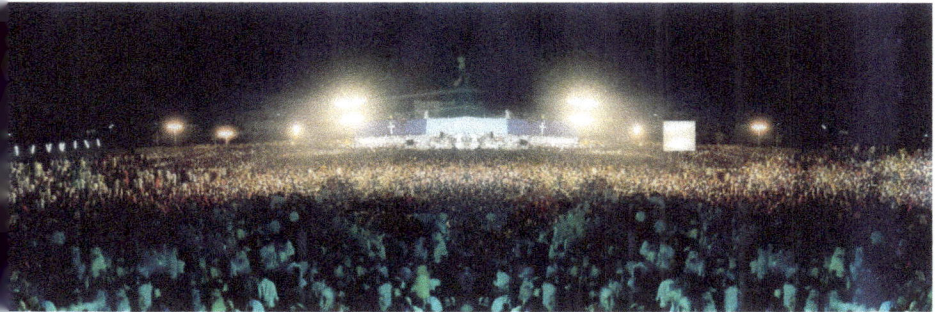

Your donations, through partnership helps us to love more, win more, reach more and do more for Jesus. Love Shaun Marler.

www.ingramcontent.com/pod-product-compliance
Lightning Source LLC
Chambersburg PA
CBHW072137020426
42334CB00018B/1843